Challenges of Aging on U.S. Families: Policy and Practice Implications

Challenges of Aging on U.S. Families: Policy and Practice Implications has been co-published simultaneously as *Marriage & Family Review*, Volume 37, Numbers 1/2 2005.

Monographic Separates from *Marriage & Family Review*

For additional information on these and other Haworth Press titles, including descriptions, tables of contents, reviews, and prices, use the QuickSearch catalog at http://www.HaworthPress.com.

Challenges of Aging on U.S. Families: Policy and Practice Implications, edited by Richard K. Caputo, PhD (Vol. 37, No. 1/2, 2005). *Examines the policy and practical implications of the aging United States population, the changes within the family structure, caregiving by various family members, and the overall economic impact.*

Parent-Youth Relations: Cultural and Cross-Cultural Perspectives, edited by Gary W. Peterson, Suzanne K. Steinmetz, and Stephan M. Wilson (Vol. 35, No. 3/4, 2003; Vol. 36, No. 1/2/3/4, 2004). *A comprehensive examination of how culture interconnects with parent-child relationships.*

Emotions and the Family, edited by Richard A. Fabes, PhD (Vol. 34, No. 1/2/3/4 2002). *"An exciting collection. The contributors insightfully unfold the nature of emotions as relational processes in marriage and parenting, and illuminate how emotional communication, competence, and regulation color family life. Chapters on siblings, stepfamilies, economic stress, and family therapy add richness to the collective portrayal of how emotions infuse marital and parent-child relationships. Scholars of marital and family life will find this a valuable resource." (Ross A. Thompson, PhD, Carl A. Happold Distinguished Professor of Psychology, University of Nebraska)*

Gene-Environment Processes in Social Behaviors and Relationships, edited by Kirby Deater-Deckard, PhD, and Stephen A. Petrill, PhD (Vol. 33, No. 1/2/3, 2002). *"During recent years there have been somewhat fruitless battles on whether family influences or peer influences are more important in children's psychological development. This book is both innovative and helpful in seeking to bring the two sets of influences together through a range of studies using twin, adoptee, and stepfamily designs to assess how genetic and environmental influences may work together in bringing about individual differences in children's emotions, behavior and especially social relationships. The different research approaches provide some new ways of thinking about, and investigating, how interpersonal relationships develop and have their effects." (Michael Rutter, MD, FRS, Professor of Developmental Psychopathology, Institute of Psychiatry, King's College, London)*

Pioneering Paths in the Study of Families: The Lives and Careers of Family Scholars, edited by Suzanne K. Steinmetz, PhD, MSW, and Gary W. Peterson, PhD (Vol. 30, No. 3, 2000; Vol. 30, No. 4, 2001; Vol. 31, No. 1/2/3/4, 2001; Vol. 32, No. 1/2, 2001). *The fascinating autobiographies of 40 leading scholars in sociology, family studies, psychology, and child development.*

FATHERHOOD: Research, Interventions and Policies, edited by H. Elizabeth Peters, PhD, Gary W. Peterson, PhD, Suzanne K. Steinmetz, PhD, MSW, and Randal D. Day, PhD (Vol. 29, No. 2/3/4, 2000). *Brings together the latest facts to help researchers explore the father-child relationship and determine what factors lead fathers to be more or less involved in the lives of their children, including human social behavior, not living with a child, being denied visiting privileges, and social norms regarding gender differences versus work responsibilities.*

Concepts and Definitions of Family for the 21st Century, edited by Barbara H. Settles, PhD, Suzanne K. Steinmetz, PhD, MSW, Gary W. Peterson, PhD, and Marvin B. Sussman, PhD (Vol. 28, No. 3/4, 1999). *Views family from a U.S. perspective and from many different cultures and societies. The controversial question "What is family?" is thoroughly examined as it has become an increasingly important social policy concern in recent years as the traditional family has changed.*

The Role of the Hospitality Industry in the Lives of Individuals and Families, edited by Pamela R. Cummings, PhD, Francis A. Kwansa, PhD, and Marvin B. Sussman, PhD (Vol. 28, No. 1/2, 1998). *"A must for human resource directors and hospitality educators." (Dr. Lynn Huffman, Director, Restaurant, Hotel, and Institutional Management, Texas Tech University, Lubbock, Texas)*

Stepfamilies: History, Research, and Policy, edited by Irene Levin, PhD, and Marvin B. Sussman, PhD (Vol. 26, No. 1/2/3/4, 1997). *"A wide range of individually valuable and stimulating chapters that form a wonderfully rich menu from which readers of many different kinds will find exciting and satisfying selections." (Jon Bernardes, PhD, Principal Lecturer in Sociology, University of Wolverhampton, Castle View Dudley, United Kingdom)*

Families and Adoption, edited by Harriet E. Gross, PhD, and Marvin B. Sussman, PhD (Vol. 25, No. 1/2/3/4, 1997). *"Written in a lucid and easy-to-read style, this volume will make an invaluable contribution to the adoption literature." (Paul Sachdev, PhD, Professor, School of Social Work, Memorial University of Newfoundland, St. John's, Newfoundland, Canada)*

The Methods and Methodologies of Qualitative Family Research, edited by Jane F. Gilgun, PhD, LICSW, and Marvin B. Sussman, PhD (Vol 24, No. 1/2/3/4, 1997). *"An authoritative look at the usefulness of qualitative research methods to the family scholar." (Family Relations)*

Intercultural Variation in Family Research and Theory: Implications for Cross-National Studies, Volumes I and II, edited by Marvin B. Sussman, PhD, and Roma S. Hanks, PhD (Vol. 22, No. 1/2/3/4, and Vol. 23, No. 1/2/3/4, 1997). *Documents the development of family research in theory in societies around the world and inspires continued cross-national collaboration on current research topics.*

Families and Law, edited by Lisa J. McIntyre, PhD, and Marvin B. Sussman, PhD (Vol. 21, No. 3/4, 1995). *With this new volume, family practitioners and scholars can begin to increase the family's position in relation to the law and legal system.*

Exemplary Social Intervention Programs for Members and Their Families, edited by David Guttmann, DSW, and Marvin B. Sussman, PhD (Vol. 21, No. 1/2, 1995). *An eye-opening look at organizations and individuals who have created model family programs that bring desired results.*

Single Parent Families: Diversity, Myths and Realities, edited by Shirley M. H. Hanson, RN, PhD, Marsha L. Heims, RN, EdD, Doris J. Julian, RN, EdD, and Marvin B. Sussman, PhD (Vol. 20, No. 1/2/3/4, 1994). *"Remarkable! . . . A significant work and is important reading for multidisciplinary family professionals including sociologists, educators, health care professionals, and policymakers." (Maureen Leahey, RN, PhD, Director, Outpatient Mental Health Program, Director, Family Therapy Training Program, Calgary District Hospital Group)*

Families on the Move: Immigration, Migration, and Mobility, edited by Barbara H. Settles, PhD, Daniel E. Hanks III, MS, and Marvin B. Sussman, PhD (Vol 19, No 1/2/3/4, 1993). *Examines the current research on family mobility, migration, and immigration and discovers new directions for understanding the relationship between mobility and family life.*

American Families and the Future: Analyses of Possible Destinies, edited by Barbara H. Settles, PhD, Roma S. Hanks, PhD, and Marvin B. Sussman, PhD (Vol. 18, No. 3/4, 1993). *This book discusses a variety of issues that face and will continue to face families in coming years and describes various strategies families can use in their decision-making processes.*

Publishing in Journals on the Family: Essays on Publishing, edited by Roma S. Hanks, PhD, Linda Matocha, PhD, RN, and Marvin B. Sussman, PhD (Vol. 18, No. 1/2, 1993). *This helpful book contains varied perspectives from scholars at different career stages and from editors of major publication outlets, providing readers with important information necessary to help them systematically plan a productive scholarly career.*

Publishing in Journals on the Family: A Survey and Guide for Scholars, Practitioners, and Students, edited by Roma S. Hanks, PhD, Linda Matocha, PhD, RN, and Marvin B. Sussman, PhD (Vol. 17, No. 3/4, 1992). *"Comprehensive. . . . Includes listings for some 200 social science journals whose editors have expressed an interest in publishing empirical research and theoretical articles about the family." (Reference & Research Book News)*

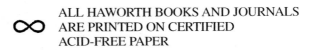

Challenges of Aging on U.S. Families: Policy and Practice Implications

Richard K. Caputo
Editor

Challenges of Aging on U.S. Families: Policy and Practice Implications has been co-published simultaneously as *Marriage & Family Review*, Volume 37, Numbers 1/2 2005.

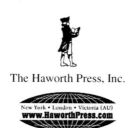

The Haworth Press, Inc.

New York • London • Victoria (AU)
www.HaworthPress.com

Challenges of Aging on U.S. Families: Policy and Practice Implications has been co-published simultaneously as *Marriage & Family Review*™, Volume 37, Numbers 1/2 2005.

The Haworth Press, Inc., 10 Alice Street, Binghamton, NY 13904-1580 USA

Cover design by Lora Wiggins

Library of Congress Cataloging-in-Publication Data

Challenges of aging on U.S. families : policy and practice implications / Richard K. Caputo, editor.
     p. cm.
"Co-published simultaneously as Marriage & family review, vol. 37, no. 1/2 2005."
Includes bibliographical references and index.
ISBN-13: 978-0-7890-2876-1 (hc. : alk. paper)
ISBN-10: 0-7890-2876-X (hc. : alk. paper)
ISBN-13: 978-0-7890-2877-8 (pbk. : alk. paper)
ISBN-10: 0-7890-2877-8 (pbk. : alk. paper)
    1. Older people–United States–Family relationships. 2. Older people–Government policy–United States. 3. Older people–Services for–United States. 4. Older people–United States–Social conditions. 5. Aging–United States. I. Caputo, Richard K.

HQ1064.U5C46 2005
305.26'0973–dc22

                      2005004038

Indexing, Abstracting & Website/Internet Coverage

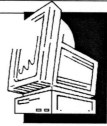

This section provides you with a list of major indexing & abstracting services and other tools for bibliographic access. That is to say, each service began covering this periodical during the year noted in the right column. Most Websites which are listed below have indicated that they will either post, disseminate, compile, archive, cite or alert their own Website users with research-based content from this work. (This list is as current as the copyright date of this publication.)

(continued)

(continued)

(continued)

   *Exact start date to come.

Special Bibliographic Notes related to special journal issues (separates) and indexing/abstracting:

- indexing/abstracting services in this list will also cover material in any "separate" that is co-published simultaneously with Haworth's special thematic journal issue or DocuSerial. Indexing/abstracting usually covers material at the article/chapter level.
- monographic co-editions are intended for either non-subscribers or libraries which intend to purchase a second copy for their circulating collections.
- monographic co-editions are reported to all jobbers/wholesalers/approval plans. The source journal is listed as the "series" to assist the prevention of duplicate purchasing in the same manner utilized for books-in-series.
- to facilitate user/access services all indexing/abstracting services are encouraged to utilize the co-indexing entry note indicated at the bottom of the first page of each article/chapter/contribution.
- this is intended to assist a library user of any reference tool (whether print, electronic, online, or CD-ROM) to locate the monographic version if the library has purchased this version but not a subscription to the source journal.
- individual articles/chapters in any Haworth publication are also available through the Haworth Document Delivery Service (HDDS).

To my wife Mary Cianni

ABOUT THE EDITOR

Richard K. Caputo is Professor of Social Policy and Research at the Wurzweiler School of Social Work, Yeshiva University, New York City. He has authored four books and numerous articles in peer-reviewed journals. Dr. Caputo serves on the editorial boards of the *Journal of Poverty*, the *Journal of Sociology & Social Welfare*, and the *Journal of Family and Economic Issues*. He is the co-recipient of the Richard A. Swanson Award for Research Excellence 1998 by the Academy of Human Resource Development. Dr. Caputo's current interests include social justice, poverty, and retirement.

Challenges of Aging on U.S. Families: Policy and Practice Implications

CONTENTS

General Editors' Comments

Richard K. Caputo was the editor for the collection of articles, "Challenges of Aging on U.S. Families: Policy and Practice Implications." This volume is most timely as the first group of baby boomers, the largest generation in U.S. history, is preparing to enter the retirement stage of their lives.

Although boomers born in the mid-to-late 1940s have done well, those born in the late 1950s to early 1960s have entered adulthood at a time when manufacturing jobs have disappeared. As a result, this group is not as likely to continue the trend of each succeeding generation experiencing a standard of living that exceeded that of their parents' generation. Most importantly, recent changes in Social Security mean that they will not only pay higher amounts of their salary into this fund, and will be required to do so beyond the traditional retirement age of 65, those born after 1960 will experience a reduction of over 30% in benefits if they retire early–defined as before the age of 67.

This impacts families at several levels. We are living longer, but this increasing life span means that we are more likely to experience longer-term illness or disability at an older age. As a result, an elderly parent may require assistance at a time when their own children are defined as elderly. Thus, it is no longer the 40-year-old child caring for the 60-year-old parent; but the child in his or her 60s caring for a parent who is 80 or older.

In order to maintain one's standard of living, the elderly are not only working longer hours, but are working beyond their 60s. At the same time, they also may be caring for still older parents as well as fulfilling the

[Haworth co-indexing entry note]: "General Editors' Comments." Steinmetz, Suzanne K., and Gary W. Peterson. Co-published simultaneously in *Marriage & Family Review* (The Haworth Press, Inc.) Vol. 37, No. 1/2, 2005, pp. 1-2; and: *Challenges of Aging on U.S. Families: Policy and Practice Implications* (ed: Richard K. Caputo) The Haworth Press, Inc., 2005, pp. 1-2. Single or multiple copies of this article are available for a fee from The Haworth Document Delivery Service [1-800-HAWORTH, 9:00 a.m. - 5:00 p.m. (EST). E-mail address: docdelivery@ haworthpress.com].

http://www.haworthpress.com/web/MFR
Digital Object Identifier: 10.1300/J002v37n01_01

role of "skipped generation parenting." Based on recent Census data, approximately 1.3 million children lived in grandparent homes where neither parent is present.

This above statistic demonstrates one of the ways in which families' structures have changed. One is likely to have not only biological parents, but also stepparents who might have legitimate claims on their adult children's resources. Families are also smaller with fewer siblings, resulting in fewer adult children, aunts, uncles, or cousins to share the caregiving tasks. And these family members are more likely than in the past to live in different parts of the country.

A reading of the articles in this collection suggests that as these baby boomers need assistance, our society will be faced with a severe labor shortage as family members are often working full-time in addition to caring for children. The stay-at-home, empty-nest wife who was available to provide care in the past is no longer a reality. Two suggestions from this collection are provided: (1) paying family caregivers so that they can leave their paid employment in order to provide this care, and (2) requiring adult children to provide care much as we require parents to care for their children. Both of these ideas will surely be controversial if they become mandated as part of the U.S. policy. Should we as a society pay family members to care for their elderly? Shouldn't they be willing to do so out of love and filial responsibility? On the other hand, should adult children be *required*, by law, to provide care for their elderly parents–which brings up some interesting moral dilemmas? Given one has a limited amount of time and money, where should that effort be put–helping one's elderly spouse, adult child or grandchildren, or helping one's aging parents?

This collection raises important policy and practice implication and provides insights into the challenges of aging that families face.

Suzanne K. Steinmetz
Gary W. Peterson
Editors
Marriage & Family Review

Editor's Introduction:
Challenges of Aging on U.S. Families:
Policy and Practice Implications

Richard K. Caputo

This volume addresses challenges of aging on families in the United States. It begins with an overview of the economic status of aging families in the U.S., then focuses primarily on two different roles that elderly family members are likely to play should contemporary aspects of family life continue over the next several decades: the formidable demands they create on caregivers and the beneficent supply of parenting resources they make available for needy grandchildren.

In the first article, Kutza examines factors that influence the economic status of families with aging household members. She pays particular attention to economic trends, public and private income maintenance policies, and marital and family relations. Although the impact of these factors on today's retirees has been mostly positive, Kutza identifies current trends that signify a retreat from the strong economic gains made by the elderly over the past 50 years. She highlights how changes in family structure and composition are likely to affect the economic status of Baby Boomers in retirement. Kutza concludes concerns about contemporary efforts to shift more responsibility from public initiatives and programs designed to minimize the prospect of aging persons falling into poverty to individuals. The remaining articles fall

[Haworth co-indexing entry note]: "Editor's Introduction: Challenges of Aging on U.S. Families: Policy and Practice Implications." Caputo, Richard K. Co-published simultaneously in *Marriage & Family Review* (The Haworth Press, Inc.) Vol. 37, No. 1/2, 2005, pp. 3-8; and: *Challenges of Aging on U.S. Families: Policy and Practice Implications* (ed: Richard K. Caputo) The Haworth Press, Inc., 2005, pp. 3-8. Single or multiple copies of this article are available for a fee from The Haworth Document Delivery Service [1-800-HAWORTH, 9:00 a.m. - 5:00 p.m. (EST). E-mail address: docdelivery@haworthpress.com].

Digital Object Identifier: 10.1300/J002v37n01_02

into two broad categories, that of caregivers and their needs, and that of grandparents raising grandchildren.

There are five articles in this collection that address various aspects of family members as caregivers meeting the needs of their aging parents. The first article, by Feld, Dunkle, and Schroepfer, examines the simultaneous effects of the health of both partners on the likelihood of solo spousal caregiving. They rely on an aging couple sub-sample of a nationally representative sample of over 8,000 community-dwelling elders, aged 70 and older, and their spouses or partners. Factors associated with expanding caregiver networks beyond the spouse include poorer health among those who needed assistance, a greater limitations with regard to Activities of Daily Living (ADL), *lengthier* marriages, and, to a lesser extent, being Black. This study provides evidence that many aging couples seek caregivers other than their spouses when needing assistance, but that longer married couples may nonetheless be less likely to do so. Family practitioners and other professionals who assess the need for outside assistance in elderly married couples are well advised to consider, among other things, the needs and desires of the couple as a unit.

Gaugler, Anderson, and Holmes review the literature in regard to existing intervention strategies designed to promote family involvement following institutionalization of an aging member. They focus in particular on two types of family-based interventions that have received scientific evaluations, namely, group-based and family-staff partnership approaches to residential long-term care. The authors identify limitations of the eleven studies that resulted from their multi-pronged literature review. These include conceptualization of family care, the lack of ethnic, racial, and socioeconomic diversity in recruited samples, sample attrition, and the a-theoretical nature of most studies. They recommend ways to overcome these limitations. They stress the importance of developing multi-component intervention approaches, such as those based on family life education (FLE) principles, identifying multiple stakeholders, and taking into account the resident's perspective when attempting to increase and facilitate family involvement in the residential care of their elders.

Li and Seltzer examine the effects of relationship strain and affective closeness with parents on daughter caregivers' self-esteem, and whether their effects are moderated by daughter role salience. Guided by identity theory and the life course perspective, their Wisconsin-based cross-sectional study of 137 married daughter caregivers with children shows that (1) relationship strain has negative effects on the daughters' self-esteem, regardless of daughter role salience, and (2) the positive effects of affective closeness on self-esteem are stronger for daughters whose daughter role is salient than for those less salient. Findings suggest that caregiving need not be viewed solely as a negative predicament. Rather, parent care offers an opportunity for daughters to improve their sense of self, as well as one that poses risk for devaluation of the self. In light of their findings, the authors discuss how practitioners can help married daughters manage relationship strain with their parents, examine the personal meaning of their daughter role, and bolster their own self-esteem while engaged in parent care.

Simon-Rusinowitz, Mahoney, Loughlin, and Sadler report findings from the Cash and Counseling Demonstration and Evaluation in Arkansas. In this demonstration, project consumers receive a cash allowance to purchase personal assistance services. Findings indicate that consumers who hired relatives received more service and had equal or superior satisfaction and health outcomes compared to those who hired non-relatives. Adding focused-group findings that help clarify and exemplify the results of the quantitative study, the authors addressed the following concerns that policymakers frequently ask: reasons consumers choose to hire relatives, who will choose to hire relatives, the impact of this consumer-directed approach on consumers, informal caregivers and paid family caregivers, as well as the quality of care provided by a relative, and concerns about fraud and abuse. They conclude that the experience of clients and their family workers are quite positive in every area of concern to policymakers that they examined.

Caputo examines the relative influence of inheritance-related and intergenerational factors on the likelihood of adult daughters providing personal care or income to their aging parents. The study sample (n = 399) is drawn from the National Longitudinal Surveys, Young Women's Cohort. Findings indicate that intergenerational factors add no explanatory power to other factors influencing the likelihood of adult daughters providing personal care for their aging parents but that inheritance-related factors do, suggesting the motivational primacy of self-interest. Also, intergenerational factors and inheritance-related factors increase the likelihood of providing financial assistance beyond that of other factors, suggesting mixed motivations, part self-interest, part social norm or altruistic, informed by the health status of the aging parents. Findings challenge the primacy of an "ethic of care" attributed to adult children in general and adult daughters in particular in regard to filial obligation to parents when it comes to providing personal care. They also in part support "ethic of care" theories when it comes to providing financial assistance. Findings suggest that targeted legislation with specific incentives may be more effective than bully pulpit or moral exhortations to ensure sufficient care by adult children for aging Baby Boomers in non-institutionalized settings for as long as possible to offset the costs of more formal care in years to come.

The final paper examining caregiving by family members authored by Chadiha, Miller-Cribbs, Rafferty, Adams, Pierce, and Kommidi report findings of an exploratory study of 251 African American female caregivers' participation in family reunions. They note that such reunions play a vital role in preserving extended families. Theirs is one of a few studies that compare urban and rural family reunions in general and in light of caregivers' participation in particular. Predictors of family reunions differed for urban and rural caregivers. Predictors of urban caregivers' participation were presence of children less than 18 years of age, having two or more other helpers compared to no helpers, and fewer chronic conditions of elders needing care. Predictors of rural caregivers' participation were positively associated with level of family functioning and inversely associated with presence of a spouse. Chadiha et al. conclude that the vitality of family reunions as sources of support to African American female caregivers must be carefully considered by service providers and they explain why this is so in light of the findings of their study. Their research provides evidence that such support may lead to more nuances in regard to future research and service delivery. Their findings provide critical baseline information on urban and rural caregivers' family reunion participation in the context of caregiving.

Three papers in this collection examine various aspects of caregiving, but it is the elder generation, the grandparents, who are providing the care to their grandchildren. Hayslip and Kaminski identify and discuss six salient issues that have come to define the study of custodial grandparents and that have implications for both researchers and practitioners: (1) theoretical and conceptual frameworks relevant to the study of custodial grandparents, (2) diversity among grandparent caregivers, (3) the importance of social support in the lives of such grandparents, (4) the impact of custodial grandparenting on relationships with others, (5) the salience of acquiring parenting skills for such grandparents, and (6) the availability and efficacy of helping interventions for grandparent caregivers. They also discuss the need for longitudinal studies to shed light on the antecedents of parental styles and coping mechanisms employed by custodial grandparents. They recommend that interventions target grandparents *and* grandchildren and they explore cultural variations in custodial grandparenting.

In their study of 133 grandparent caregivers with full-time responsibility of raising at least one grandchild, Landry-Meyer, Gerard, and Guzell show that caregiver stress (measured by the Parental Stress Index) is associated negatively with life satisfaction (measured by the Life Satisfaction Index-Z) and generativity (i.e., active engagement in life measured by the Loyola Generativity Scale). Informal and formal social supports (e.g., social networks, perceived support, and enacted support) have a beneficial influence on stress outcomes that generalizes to grandparent caregiver participants regardless of the amount of stress they experience. Contrary to predictions based on stress theory, however, Landry-Meyer, Gerard, and Guzell report that social support does not buffer the association between caregiver stress and life satisfaction nor between caregiver stress and generativity. They speculate that while network members provide needed support to grandparents, they may also be a constant reminder that grandparent caregivers are off-time with same-age peers. Connections with friends and family who are engaged in on-time and better-rewarded paths to generativity may lead grandparent caregivers to feel like their contribution to society is less important especially with the increased stress associated with re-parenting. Findings lend to grandparent caregivers' perceived need for social services. Such services provide generational continuity when caregivers can no longer rely on support they once received from informal support network.

Using data from the National Survey of America's Families, Mills, Gomez-Smith, and De Leon examine factors associated with the frequency of feelings of psychosocial distress among grandmother caregivers of grandchildren in skipped generation families. Findings indicate that for these grandmothers, being Black and living in the Midwest, having a family income below the poverty level, having Medicaid or SCHIP coverage, not receiving Welfare payments for childcare, and having a usual place for health care are all associated with more frequent feelings of psychosocial distress. On the other hand, being married, receiving social services help with childcare, grandmother's perception of less parenting burden, and living below poverty in the Midwest are associated with less frequent feelings of psychosocial distress. They conclude that the importance of psychological counseling for grandparents who raise grandchildren without benefit of the children's parents is nonetheless clear. Mills, Gomez-Smith, and De Leon recommend that social services and health providers can play an important role in helping these grandmothers to overcome barriers, such as fear of stigma, financial cost, or lack of information about available services. They also recommend that more favorable consideration must be given to public assistance for caregiving grandparents, especially to poor women who are more likely to be the caregivers in skipped generation households. It is imperative that more policy makers acknowledge the social good accomplished by these women caregivers who are struggling to keep their families intact despite incredible barriers.

This collection provides insights into the economic and caregiving problems that will be faced by a relatively large group of individuals, the Baby Boomers, over the next several decades. It also demonstrates that not only are aging grandparents likely to need care, many are finding themselves in a position where they are called upon to care for their grandchildren. As the articles in this volume show, scholars have begun to address these issues and offer fruitful considerations for policy makers and others concerned with the impact of aging on families in the U.S.

I wish to acknowledge the following individuals who served on the Editorial Board for this project:

Charles Auerbach, Yeshiva University-Wilf Campus
Catherine Goodman, California State University, Long Beach
Miriam Dinerman, Yeshiva University-Wilf Campus
Margaret Gibelman, Yeshiva University-Wilf Campus
Martha Ozawa, Washington University
Betty Sancier, University of Wisconsin-Milwaukee
Roberta G. Sands, University of Pennsylvania
Sharron Singleton, Barry University
Barry Trute, McGill University
Thomas Young, Widener University

The Intersection of Economics and Family Status in Late Life: Implications for the Future

Elizabeth A. Kutza

SUMMARY. The factors that influence economic status in late life are examined with particular attention to economic trends, public and private income maintenance policies, and marital and family relations. While the impact of these factors on today's retirees has been mostly positive, current trends are identified that may result in a retreat from the strong economic gains made by the elderly over the past 50 years. An examination of how changes in family structure and composition may affect the economic status of Baby Boomers in retirement is highlighted. *[Article copies available for a fee from The Haworth Document Delivery Service: 1-800-HAWORTH. E-mail address: <docdelivery@haworthpress.com> Website: <http://www.HaworthPress.com> © 2005 by The Haworth Press, Inc. All rights reserved.]*

KEYWORDS. Economic security, Baby Boomers, retirement income, U.S. social policy

Elizabeth A. Kutza is Professor of Community Health and Director, Institute on Aging, Portland State University, Urban Center, Room 470P, Portland, OR 97201 (E-mail: kutzae@pdx.edu).

[Haworth co-indexing entry note]: "The Intersection of Economics and Family Status in Late Life: Implications for the Future." Kutza, Elizabeth A. Co-published simultaneously in *Marriage & Family Review* (The Haworth Press, Inc.) Vol. 37, No. 1/2, 2005, pp. 9-26; and: *Challenges of Aging on U.S. Families: Policy and Practice Implications* (ed: Richard K. Caputo) The Haworth Press, Inc., 2005, pp. 9-26. Single or multiple copies of this article are available for a fee from The Haworth Document Delivery Service [1-800-HAWORTH, 9:00 a.m. - 5:00 p.m. (EST). E-mail address: docdelivery@haworthpress.com].

http://www.haworthpress.com/web/MFR
© 2005 by The Haworth Press, Inc. All rights reserved.
Digital Object Identifier: 10.1300/J002v37n01_03

In June of 1934, President Franklin Delano Roosevelt sent a message to Congress outlining what the nation needed to do as it tried to recover from the Great Depression. He noted that individuals and their families then, much as now, wanted three things in their lives–a decent home to live in, productive work, and "some safeguards against misfortunes which cannot be wholly eliminated in the man-made world of ours" (*Report of the Committee on Economic Security*, 1985, p. 1). By Executive Order, Roosevelt created a Committee on Economic Security to make recommendations to him concerning this third desire of the citizenry. These recommendations resulted in the passage of the Social Security Act (1935) and the implementation of a key element of economic security for future elderly, Old Age Survivors Insurance (OASI).

But economic status in late life is not only influenced by public income maintenance policies, but also by broad economic trends, one's personal work history, and one's family structure. Since the passage of the Social Security Act, the nation has experienced several economic fluctuations, i.e., periods of relatively short recessions followed by periods of sustained economic growth. There also have been social changes in American society including a rise in the average level of education, a shift from a manufacturing to a service economy, increased participation of women in the labor force, and changing family structures. The impact these changes have had on today's retirees has been mostly positive. But current trends can be identified that may result in a retreat from the strong economic gains made by the elderly over the past 50 years. For the Baby Boomer cohorts and those that follow them, economic security in old age may become more fragile.

Since the end of World War II, our nation has experienced a period of sustained economic growth thus allowing most Americans to enjoy a higher standard of living than would have been possible a generation earlier. Between 1949 and 1959, for example, median family income grew by 43% and, by 1960, there was one car for every 1.8 adults (Levy, 1998). From 1940 to 1958, the size of the U.S. economy (in real terms) doubled and it doubled again in the next 20 years (Friedland & Summer, 1999). Current retirees have benefited from this economic growth as evidenced by their asset position. The median net worth of persons aged 65 to 74 in 2000 was $146,500 and 81% of this age group owned their own home. Of those aged 75 and older, 77% own their own homes and have an average net worth of $125,000 (U.S. Census Bureau, 2000, Table 763). These assets can cushion any loss of income sustained in retirement.

Today's retirees are also the first cohort of workers to begin their careers as contributors to social security. And, for the bulk of their careers, their contributions coincided with a period of dramatic growth in real wages. The Old Age Survivors Insurance (OASI) provisions under the Social Security Act allocates monthly cash benefits to individual Americans who have reached a designated "old age" and who have made contributions to the Social Security System through payroll taxes. Benefits are based upon the insured worker's average monthly earnings in covered employment. The benefit formula is explicitly redistributive with low wage workers receiving higher benefits in relation to their past earnings than do workers with high average earnings. At the time of retirement, the formula takes into account wage inflation; after retirement, monthly benefits are adjusted for price inflation. As Aaron and his colleagues note (Aaron, Bosworth, & Burtless, 1989), the OASI program "has been conspicuously successful in raising the income of elderly and disabled Americans . . . the steady increase in benefits has reduced the percentage of elderly and disabled Americans living in poverty" (p. 31). Poverty among the elderly has declined substantially during the past 35 years. In 1967, 30% of persons over the age of 65 had incomes below the federal poverty level (U.S. Bureau of the Census, 1998). By 2001, the poverty rate for this age group was 10.1% (U.S. Bureau of the Census, 2003).

In addition to benefiting from sustained economic growth and enhancements in the social security program, persons now in retirement worked during a period of rapid expansion of private pension plans. It was not until the 1940s and 1950s that employer-provided private pension schemes began to take hold. Analysts attribute this growth to several factors–wage freezes during World War II and the Korean War that encouraged fringe benefit growth in lieu of wages, inducements in the Internal Revenue tax code, union activism, and a decision by the National Labor Relations Board that pensions were a proper issue for collective bargaining (Schulz, 2001). As a consequence of these factors, the total number of workers covered under private pension plans increased from 12% of private wage and salary labor force in 1940 to about 45% in 1990 (U.S. Department of Labor, 1993). Workers in high pay and unionized industries and occupations are most likely to be employed by firms sponsoring plans, as are workers who are college graduates. Service industry workers, who now make up almost one-third of the private sector wage and salary labor force, are least likely to be employed in a firm sponsoring a pension plan (U.S. Department of Labor, 2003).

As a result of these three economic trends–(1) sustained economic growth, (2) enhancements in Old Age Survivors Insurance benefits, and (3) expansion of private pensions–individuals who reached their 60s in the mid-to-latter part of the 20th century were able to exit the workforce with considerable financial stability and security. Retirement became an option, not a forced choice. Until the 1970s, most labor force decline in late life was involuntary. Only a very small percentage of retired men reported leaving work because they wanted to retire. Prior to the passage of the Age Discrimination in Employment Act (ADEA) of 1967, mandatory retirement rules explained much of this decline with the rest attributed to poor health (Ozawa & Law, 1992; Quinn, 1999) or involuntary layoffs.

More recently, however, older workers report leaving the labor market because of a desire for more leisure. As Hardy (2002) aptly notes: "The latter part of the twentieth century may well by remembered as the 'era of retirement,' since it was during the final few decades that this stage became an expected and usually welcome part of the life course" (p. 9). It might be more accurate, however, to call this period the "golden age of retirement," one not likely to be experienced by the children of current retirees who are in the Baby Boom generation.

FAMILY DETERMINANTS OF WELL-BEING

Family composition, family size, and family role obligations also have an impact on an individual's economic security in late life. For example, the association between marital status and economic security in old age is well documented, especially as it affects women. Poverty rates for the elderly are highest among divorced, never married, and widowed women. Compared to 4.4% of married elderly women, 20.3% of divorced, 16.5% of widowed, and 23.1% of never-married elderly women are living in poverty. More than half of elderly widows now living in poverty were not poor before the death of their husbands (U.S. Department of Health and Human Services, 2001).

Although labor force participation of women has increased over the past 50 years (in 1940, women made up 24% of the total labor force; by the mid-90s, that figure was 46%), throughout their lives women must still reconcile their family responsibilities with their work roles. For example, women spend, on average, 12 years out of the work force for family caregiving over the course of their lives, whether for children, a spouse, and/or parents (OWL, 2002). When in the workforce, many women choose part-time jobs so as to continue to meet their familial responsibilities. Twenty-six percent of women workers are employed on a part-time basis compared to only 12% of male workers, which affects income status both during midlife and in retirement. Pension coverage rates for part-time employees are only 14% compared to 51% for those employed full time (U.S. Department of Labor, 2003). In fact, pension plans are permitted to exclude workers who work less than 1,000 hours per year so even if a woman works in a firm with a pension plan, as a part-time employee she may be excluded from participation.

Almost from the inception of the social security program, this association between marital status and economic security in old age was recognized. Eligibility for spousal benefits, which were introduced with the 1939 Amendments to the Social Security Act (Social Security Act Amendments, 1939) was an acknowledgement of the social and economic functions of the family (McNamara, O'Grady-LeShane, & Williamson, 2003). Women were presumed to marry. The state of marriage in the 1930s presumed a sole economic dependency upon the husband and a full-time commitment to homemaking. Even today, most federal economic policies whether concerning taxation, social security, or pension reform, regard women as dependents of their husbands. Hence, even without husband through divorce or death, a woman's benefits under an income maintenance policy are defined relative to the absent husband.

The 1939 Social Security dependent and survivor benefits continue to be important for women in terms of their economic security in retirement. Although women have progressed economically in recent decades due to greater labor force participation, they continue to be more dependent on Social Security benefits than men. Significant percentages of unmarried older women rely on Social Security as their sole source of retirement income. The rates are as follows—unmarried women of all races (26%), white women (24%), African American women (45%), and Latinas (46%). In contrast, Social Security provides 90% or more of income for only 19% of older married white couples and 28% of older married African American couples (OWL, 2002).

Under the dependency provisions of Old Age Insurance, women may receive benefits based upon their own or their husband's earnings record, whichever is higher. In many cases, a spousal benefit based upon 50% of a husband's prior earnings (the dependent benefit) is larger than a benefit based upon 100% of the woman's prior earnings (a primary worker benefit). While the proportion of women receiving benefits as a dependent of their husband has been declining, it represented 35% of women aged 62 and older receiving benefits in 1999 (Social Security Administration, 2000).

Thus, marriage and family patterns remain important predictors of economic security in late life especially for women. And changing family structures may have significant impacts on future generations of older persons.

THE NEW REALITY FOR BABY BOOMERS

The changing demographics of the American population have been well documented. The number of older persons in American society is growing. In 2000, 35 million people 65 years of age and over were counted by the U.S. Census Bureau. This represents a 12% increase since 1990 (Meyer, 2001). America is also getting older. During the 1990s, the most rapid growth of the older population was among those over 85 years of age (a 38% increase between 1990 and 2000) (Meyer, 2001). These trends will continue into the mid-21st century as the Baby Boom generation, those born between 1946 and 1964, reach late life. Between 2006 and 2030, the majority of Baby Boomers will enter the "young-old age groups" (60 to 75), and this age group will be nearly twice as large in 2030 as now (Morgan, 1998).

When members of the Baby Boom generation begin to retire, they will have the same needs as current retirees–a steady stream of replacement income to pay for living and healthcare expenses and a plan for how and where they want to live out their retirement years. But in many ways, the Baby Boom generation has faced a different economic environment from that of earlier generations. From the start of their work lives, this generation has experienced considerable economic fluctuation. Between 1870 and 1973, the U.S. economy grew at an average rate of 3.4% a year, excluding the effects of inflation. But between 1973 and 1993, the average rate of growth flattened to 2.3% a year (inflation adjusted) (Madrick, 1995). It was during this period that individuals born during the latter years of the Baby Boom were entering the labor force while those at the front end of the boom were nearing age 50, having spent their entire work history in a period of falling, not rising, wage levels. These levels especially fell for high school and minority workers (Madrick, 1995).

Even a college education has not saved the Baby Boomers from this downturn. The economy simply could not absorb the large number of college-educated Baby Boomers who entered the job market in the

1970s. The rate of return on a college degree, based on the salaries the graduates were getting, fell to post-war lows in these years (Freeman, 1976).

Between 1990 and 1998, personal income remained stagnant, growing at an annual rate of 2.2%. Then briefly, the economy heated up and the rate of growth for personal income doubled to 4.4% (U.S. Census Bureau, 2000). Individual savings, as represented through money market fund shares, mutual fund shares, and pension fund reserves, also grew substantially during 1999. But this economic boom was short lived. By 2003, most economic indicators were down. Stock prices were in decline, the Consumer Confidence Index was dropping, household income was 2.2% lower than in 2000 in real terms and, after falling for four consecutive years, the poverty rate rose from 11.3% in 2000 to 11.7% in 2001 (U.S. Census Bureau, 2003).

There are several consequences to this decline in the growth of worker incomes that may adversely affect the economic security of Baby Boomers in retirement. One is the effect that lowered earnings will have on future Social Security benefits. Since retirement benefits are related to pre-retirement earning levels, a lowered income stream across a work life will translate to lower benefits in retirement. Baby Boomers are not doing as well financially as their parents did in their prime work years; they will not do as well as their parents are now doing in retirement. They also will have to work longer before they receive their full Social Security benefits. Between 2000 and 2022, the "normal" age of retirement under Social Security will rise from 65 to 67. While an individual can still elect to take early retirement benefits between ages 62 and 64, the permanent, actuarial benefit reduction that accompanies this decision will become steeper. In 1999, more than half of the benefits awarded were to retirees who began receiving Social Security benefits at age 62, despite this benefit reduction (Social Security Administration, 2000). Butrica, Smith, and Toder (2002) estimate that early retirees in the 2020 population will have their benefits reduced by as much as 28.3% and those born in 1960 or later will have their benefits reduced by as much as 30% as a result of Social Security's changes in the normal retirement age. "These results," they conclude, "suggest that the reduction in the current law Social Security replacement rate will push a greater proportion of individuals with the lowest incomes below the poverty line" (p. 32). In addition, real and inflation-induced income increases will push a significant number of Baby Boomers into the range where their Social Security benefits become taxable.

A second result is that the Baby Boom generation may be saving less and borrowing more than their parents. The contention that Boomers are under-saving has been advanced most notably by Bernheim (1993, 1997), who has estimated that Boomers save on average only about one-third as much as they will need to maintain their pre-retirement standard of living. Yet, Gist, Wu and Ford (1999) caution that no study has yet measured Boomers' actual savings adequacy because an accurate assessment depends greatly on assumptions affecting resources (e.g., pension coverage, inflation, rates of return on investments) as well as a number of factors affecting needs (e.g., longevity, health costs, ability to work, and possibly costs of caregiving).

Nonetheless, Baby Boomers themselves report minimal savings for retirement and many are concerned about how they will manage. In 1997, for example, the Public Agenda Foundation surveyed 1,200 working Americans, aged 22 to 61, about retirement. The survey revealed that 38% of Baby Boomers aged 33 to 50 years old have saved less than $10,000 for retirement. Sixty-six percent of this group says they do not want to worry so much about saving for their retirement that they end up not enjoying their lives now. While these Boomers admit that they are compulsive spenders and do not save enough for retirement, few say they will change their behavior (Public Agenda Foundation, 1997). On the other hand, 41% of individuals participating in a Texas Baby Boomer survey reported concern about how they will live on their retirement savings and 40% worried that they won't be able to afford to retire. Over two-thirds (68%) said they planned to continue working after age 65 (Texas Department of Aging, 2000).

Finally, the instability in the economy in recent years has impacted the extent to which, and the way in which, private employers provide pension benefits. Over the past three decades, there has been a steady increase in pension receipt although there are still large differences in what might be called "class of worker." Government workers have higher rates than private sector employees (80% to 50%); and private employees working full-time have higher rates than those working part-time (54% to 20%). There is even a difference in coverage between early Boomers (those born in the 1946-55 period) and late Boomers (those born between 1956 and 1965). Among late Boomers, 47% reported coverage on their primary jobs–9 percentage points less than the older Boomers (Woods, 1994).

But of more significance is that important changes are occurring in the *types* of employer-sponsored retirement coverage available to workers, changes that are already having important implications for people nearing retirement and those in the Baby Boom generation. The shift is from traditional pension plans–defined benefit plans–to defined contribution plans, and more specifically, to a particular type of defined contribution plan, 401(k) plans. In a defined benefit plan, an annuity of a certain amount is guaranteed the retiree by the company. The benefit amount is usually calculated on the basis of past contributions, years of work, and the like, and it is guaranteed over the life of the retiree. In defined contribution plans, retirement benefits depend on what the person has contributed over his or her work life, as well as what the employer has matched, plus interest on those contributions. The resultant amount is all that is available in retirement, regardless of how long one lives and how one's needs may change. In 1985, 26% of full-time workers in medium and large private establishments participated in defined contribution plans, compared with 80% in defined benefit plans. By 1993, the figures were 42% and 56% (Foster, 1996).

As this trend continues, Baby Boomers in defined contribution plans face uncertain outcomes as regards their retirement funds. First, market fluctuations, such as those experienced in the late '90s and early 2000s can play havoc with one's retirement planning. After years of exuberant growth, both the recently retired and those nearing retirement are seeing their investment portfolios drop precipitously. By the end of 2002, the average 401(k) investor was back to where he or she would have been in mid-1997 (Learning painful lessons of the 401[k], 2003).

The collapse of major corporations in the late 1990s (e.g., Enron, Global Crossing, WorldCom, Lucent Technologies, Qwest Communications International, and Tyco) also adversely affects the retirement prospects of many Baby Boomers. The bankruptcy of one company alone, Enron, resulted in pension fund losses of over $1.5 billion. In Ohio, the state's two pension funds for government employees lost $114 million, while a California pension fund for teachers lost $49 million and New York City's fund for fire fighters, police officers, teachers, and other workers lost $109 million (Retirement funds lose 1.5 billion due to Enron fall, 2002). As large as these losses are, these public pensions are defined benefit plans so business investment failures such as those noted above may put pressure on the pension fund, but won't alter the lifetime guarantee of currently vested workers.

In contrast, the risk of loss rests entirely on the employee in defined contribution plans like 401(k)s. Consider the employees of Enron who, before the company declared bankruptcy, received 50 cents worth of Enron shares for each dollar they contributed to their 401(k) account up to 6% of their salaries. Between 2000 and 2001, Enron's falling stock prices wiped out about $1.3 billion in retirement savings of Enron employees. WorldCom employees experienced a $1.1 million loss in their company's 401(k) plan between the beginning of 2000 and the time the company filed for bankruptcy in July of 2001, while Global Crossing's pension fund losses amounted to $275 million (The 401[k] problem, 2002). Unfortunately, once these pension funds default on their obligation to their workers, there is no financial protection even for the vested worker. The Federal Pension Guarantee Trust Corporation, a creation of the 1974 Employee Retirement Income Security Act (ERISA), only insures pension benefits under defined benefit plans, not defined contribution plans.

Another blow to workers in 401(k) plans is the recent trend of companies that are facing a downturn in their profits but are remaining in business to stop matching contributions to their employees' retirement plans, thus reducing the value of the pension for the covered worker (Schwab joins others ending contributions to 401[k]s, 2003).

Finally, Baby Boomers who have lost their jobs in this recent recession have been cashing out all or some of their pension assets rather than rolling them over into their new job's plan or an Individual Retirement Account (IRA). In 2002, 22.5% of 401(k) distributions were cashed out, up from 20.2% in 2000 (Learning painful lessons of the 401[k], 2003). This short-term gain can result in long-term losses for one's portfolio at retirement.

Thus, the economic trends and policy changes of the past few decades are conspiring to leave the Baby Boom generation with more economic uncertainty in retirement. Two legs of the "three-legged stool" of financial security in retirement–savings and private pensions–are wobbly. And the third leg, Social Security, while remaining strong, is threatened by recent attempts to privatize it, thus weakening its benefit guarantee and making it more vulnerable to market fluctuations.

Proposals to partially privatize Social Security have been part of serious political debate since the mid-1990s when the 1994-1996 Advisory Council on Social Security gave major attention to Social Security financing issues and the desirability of some form of privatization. One of the most common approaches to partial privatization would require workers to pay a portion of their Social Security contribution into 401(k)-like individual Social Security Retirement Accounts (Advisory Council on Social Security, 1997). Several arguments have been put forward in support of such privatization. Proponents argue that privatization will increase the rate of economic growth, increase the rate of return on Social Security contributions, and help protect Baby Boomers against sharp reductions in their Social Security benefits. In his critique of privatization, however, Williamson (1997) notes, "Even if a privatization scheme is designed so as to give a substantial boost to the American economy and to ensure that the average worker would be better off than under the current social security scheme, it is possible that many workers, particularly low-wage workers, would end up worse" (p. 569). More recent analyses point to the detrimental effect privatization would have on older women (OWL, 2002). More than any other group, women count on Social Security as the primary source of their retirement income. Without it, 52% of white women, 65% of African American women, and 61% of Latinas over the age of 65 would be poor (Center on Budget and Policy Priorities, 2000). Recent market declines, business failures, and 401(k) plan insolvencies have weakened the claims of privatization adherents but not silenced them (Williamson, 2002).

In sum, then, the Baby Boom generation may find that contrary to their parents' expectation and experience of the government as the provider of a floor of protection against the contingencies of old age, they will be asked to bear the associated risks of these contingencies by themselves.

THE ECONOMICALLY AT-RISK

While the Baby Boom cohort, as a group, may expect less financial certainty in retirement than earlier groups, there remains substantial diversity of financial prospects within this group. Cutler (1998) argues that there is a risk of "gero-simplification" when all members of an age group are described as similar. He directs our attention to the diversity of the Boomer generation rather than their similarities–diversity of age (nineteen years separate the early Boomers from the late Boomers), diversity in family structure, and diversity of financial status. Those with a good education, steady employment, coverage in a defined-benefit employer-sponsored pension plan, adequate savings and investments, and who are in a stable marital relationship will face a comfortable retirement. But, people "who have lacked access to education, who have experienced erratic work histories, and who are ineligible for entitlement privileges are economically at risk during the retirement phase of their lives" (Stanford & Usita, 2002, p. 45). These problems fall disproportionately on older people of color and women.

For both people of color and women, Social Security is by far the most important source of total income in retirement (Choi, 1997; OWL, 2002). This is because they receive proportionately less income from pensions, savings, and investments than white Americans. In 2001, a woman age 65 and older was only 62% as likely to receive an annuity and/or employment-based pension payment as her male counterpart. If she did receive one, her average benefit was likely to be 57% of that received by a man in the same age group (EBRI, 2003)

People of color and women also represent a disproportionate share of private household workers and farm workers, two groups of workers who may be susceptible to employers failing to report wages fully (Kijakazi, 2002). Failure to report these wages can leave some workers unable to qualify for Social Security benefits or may diminish the base upon which their Social Security benefits are calculated.

And early forecasts are that many of tomorrow's female Social Security beneficiaries will be no better off than retired women now. The Social Security Administration projects that the poverty rate for older women receiving Social Security benefits in 2020 will be the same as it was in 1991 (12%), that poverty rates will stay high (22%) among divorced women, and that poverty among never-married women will increase from 23% to 35% (Smeeding, Estes, & Glasse, 2000).

Compounding these financial disadvantages as regards retirement income, people of color more frequently than whites retire early for involuntary reasons. Diminished job opportunities and poor health in later years are crucial determinants of labor force withdrawal for these groups (Boaz, 1988). Black people, aged 51 to 59, who are retired, are less physically healthy than white people of the same age who are retired. Among young retirees, over one-third (36%) of whites report that they are in excellent to very good physical health, compared to 13% of blacks (National Academy on an Aging Society, 2000).

The combination of race and gender in old age has been referred to as a "double jeopardy" in one's risk of financial security in late life. In comparison to other minorities and white women, African American women are most likely to have been employed in jobs without pension plans, to provide care for adult children and grandchildren and to work in low-paying jobs (SPRY Foundation and National Committee to Preserve Social Security and Medicare, 1999). For Baby Boomers of color and women, then, financial insecurity in retirement may remain as problematic tomorrow as it is today.

CHANGING FAMILY STRUCTURES

At the same time that the next generation of older persons may have to shoulder more responsibility for their financial security in retirement, another source of support in old age is also changing–the family. Bould (1993) notes "An ideal-type family consisting of a husband, wife, and children living together has dominated the sociological imagination as well as social policy perspective since the New Deal" (p. 133). But this "ideal-type family" has declined in the past half century. In 1960, 88% of children lived in a two-parent household; in 1998, only 68% did. Of the remaining 32%, four-fifths lived with only one parent (usually a mother), and in 56% of these households, no other adult was present (U.S. Census Bureau, 1999).

The traditional image of family as husband, wife, and children is also being challenged by the rise in the number of childless couples. About 42% of today's families are married couples without children. The percentage of U.S. women not having children has doubled since the late 1970s, to about one in five according to the Census Bureau. In 1998, 19% of women aged 40 to 44 had not given birth to a child compared to 10% two decades earlier. For some of these women, childlessness is a deliberate choice. Others find themselves unmarried in their forties because they concentrated on their education or careers only now to be unable to find a suitable mate. But roughly one-half of these women are married and would like to have a child, but have been unable to conceive because of age-related fertility problems (Bachu, 2000). Increasingly, then, family may be characterized as two adults who have no children.

Thus, in the last century, we have seen family structures that diverge from the "ideal." Fewer families consist of a husband, wife, and their biological children living together. There are now more single-parent families, blended families, childless families, and fewer families all together.

IMPLICATIONS FOR AN AGING SOCIETY

The implications of changing family structures and roles in an aging society are several. Historically, the family has been an important institution in both the care of their children and in the care of adult family members who may be infirm or disabled. Prior to the Social Security Act and the widespread availability of public financial support in old age, children provided financial as well as physical support for their aged relatives. The family's responsibility for support of its elderly members has changed over the generations shaped by culture, modernization, changing social arrangements, and public policies. In most western industrialized societies today, this responsibility has shifted from economic support to emotional and instrumental support.

Sustained economic growth since the end of World War II has allowed current retirees to acquire their own homes and other financial assets. Public income maintenance programs such as Old Age Survivors Insurance (OASI) supplemented by private employee-sponsored pension plans have reduced the need for financial transfers from adult children to their elderly kin. In fact, by 1988, nearly twice as many older persons reported giving money to a child on a regular basis than reported receiving such support. For older persons with at least one living child, nearly one quarter gave regular financial help to their children while only 15.4% received such assistance (Freedman, Wolf, Soldo, & Stephen, 1991).

Today, intergenerational support is primarily reflected in caregiving activities rather than financial transfers. Families today provide the majority of care for dependent elders (Doty, 1995). Several trends noted above may contribute to the declining ability of families to continue to provide intensive caregiving services to their elderly relatives while at the same time adding some pressure to help if their parents' retirement income is insufficient to their needs.

First, widespread marital dissolution and smaller families result in fewer kin upon whom to rely. The fertility rate for Baby Boom cohorts, for example, is generally less than two children, compared with a rate of between 2.4 and 3.6 children in their parents' cohort (Barusch, 2000). And, as women delay childbearing, the proportion that faces the dual responsibility of caring for an elderly parent and a minor child may increase. In addition, such delays in childbearing may diminish a family's preparation for retirement. Instead of having an "empty nest" between the ages of 50 and 60 years, the peak earning period when discretionary income may be put toward retirement savings, families waiting to start their families until their 30s and even 40s will be facing college expenses for their children when they are very near to retirement.

The policy lag that now exists between the image of family extant in policy and the reality of changing family structures and norms need special attention in our aging society. As more Americans live into late old age and their needs for care and/or financial assistance increase, we can no longer assume that family members will be available or able to fill this role.

CONCLUSION

While there is some risk associated with predicting the future circumstances of the Baby Boom generation, and keeping in mind Cutler's (1998) caution of "gero-simplification," certain recent events and trends suggest concern. The first wave of the Baby Boom generation to reach retirement age will do so within the next decade. If their retirement funds were invested in securities either through money market funds or through their 401(k) plans, they may not be able to recover from losses experienced during the recession of the 2000-2003 period. If they were employed by one of the countless firms that filed for bankruptcy during this recession, their pension contributions may be lost almost completely. Even those who continue to contribute to a solvent defined contribution, employer-sponsored pension plan face the reality that their retirement income is dependent upon the swings of the market.

For those among the Baby Boom generation who will reach retirement age later in the 21st century, they may recover from any market fluctuations that are occurring today, but decisions in the public policy arena may begin to compromise their financial security in retirement. One trend on the national policy horizon which will have an impact has already been identified–the trend of government to shift responsibility for Hudson's (1993) "social contingencies" of old age from the collective to the individual. Proposed changes in Old Age Insurance and Medicare will compromise the very nature of these programs that have provided universal benefits by pooling the risks of events like unemployment, disability, and old age across the whole population. These changes will especially disadvantage people of color and women. And as the proportion of retirees to working age adults increases, the politics of intergenerational exchanges will clearly focus public discussions on intergenerational equity.

For future elderly, as for today's older persons, marital and family relations remain a critical factor in both economic security and personal coping. The capacity of families in the future to compensate for the deficiencies of public retirement policies and employer-sponsored pensions is uncertain. Smaller families and increasing rates of childlessness make reliance on family support for the Baby Boom cohort unrealistic. Poverty rates for divorced and never-married older women are projected to increase rather than decrease in 2020 when the Baby Boomers begin to retire. And as longevity for women continues to outpace the life expectancy of men, more widows will make up future cohorts of the aged. While social trends as regards marriage and the family are difficult to direct, it is imperative that public income maintenance policies attend to these changes and develop in a manner that will protect those whose income security is most affected by these trends.

REFERENCES

Aaron, H. J., Bosworth, B. P., & Burtless, G. (1989). *Can America afford to grow old? Paying for social security.* Washington, D.C.: The Brookings Institution.

Advisory Council on Social Security (1997). *Report of the 1994-1996 Advisory Council on Social Security. Volume I: Findings and recommendations.* Washington, D.C.: U.S. Government Printing Office.

Bachu, A. (2000). *Fertility of American women.* Washington, D.C.: U.S. Census Bureau.

Barusch, A. S. (2000). Social security is not for babies: Trends and policies affecting older women in the United States. *Families in Society: the Journal of Contemporary Human Services, 81,* 568-575.

Bernheim, B. D. (1993). *Is the baby boom generation preparing adequately for retirement?* (Summary report). Princeton, NJ: Merrill Lynch.

Bernheim, B. D. (1997). The adequacy of personal retirement savings: Issues and options. In D.Wise (Ed.), *Facing the age wave* (pp. 30-56). Stanford, CA: Hoover Institution Press.

Boaz, R. F. (1988). Early withdrawal from the labor force: A response only to pension pull or also to labor market push? *Research on Aging, 9,* 530-547.

Bould, S. (1993). Familial caretaking: A middle-range definition of family in the context of social policy. *Journal of Family Issues, 14,* 133-151.

Butrica, B. A., Smith, K., & Toder, E. (2002, September). *Projecting poverty rates in 2020 for the 62 and older population: What changes can we expect and why?* (Working paper 2002-3). Chestnut Hill, MA: Center for Retirement Research at Boston College.

Center on Budget and Policy Priorities (2000). Social security reform and women of color. Presentation by Kilolo Kijakazi, February.

Choi, N. G. (1997). Racial differences in retirement income: The roles of public and private income sources. *Journal of Aging & Social Policy, 9*(3), 21-42.

Cutler, N. E. (1998). Preparing for their older years: The financial diversity of aging boomers. *Generations, 22*(1), 81-86.

Doty, P. (1995). Family care of the elderly: The role of public policy. *Milbank Memorial Fund Quarterly, 64,* 34-75.

EBRI (2003). *Retirement annuity and employment-based pension income.* (January Notes). Washington, D.C.: Employee Benefit Research Institute.

Foster, A. C. (1996). Employee participation in savings and thrift plans, 1993. *Monthly Labor Review, 119*(3), 17-22.

Freedman, V. A., Wolf, D. A., Soldo, B. J., & Stephen, E. H. (1991). Intergenerational transfers: A question of perspective. *The Gerontologist, 31*, 640-647.

Freeman, R. (1976). *The overeducated American.* New York: Academic Press.

Friedland, R. B. & Summer, L. (1999). Demography is not destiny. Washington, D.C.: National Academy on an Aging Society, The Gerontological Society of America.

Gist, J. R., Wu, K. B., & Ford, C. (1999). *Do baby boomers save and, if so, what for?* AARP Public Policy Institute (#9906), Washington, D.C.: American Association of Retired Persons.

Hardy, M. A. (2002). The transformation of retirement in twentieth-century America: From discontent to satisfaction. *Generations, 26*(11), 9-16.

Hudson, R. B. (1999). "Social contingencies, the aged, and public policy." *The Milbank Quarterly, 71*, 253-277.

Kijakazi, K. (2002). Impact of unreported social security earnings on people of color and women. *Public Policy and Aging Report, 12*(3), 9-12. Washington, D.C.: Gerontological Society of America.

Learning painful lessons of the 401(k). (2003, March 18). *The New York Times*, p. E11.

Levy, F. (1998). *The new dollars and dreams: American incomes and economic change.* New York: Russell Sage Foundation.

Madrick, J. (1995). *The end of affluence.* New York: Random House.

McNamara, T. K., O'Grady-LeShane, R., & Williamson, J. B. (2003). *The role of marital history, early retirement benefits, and the economic status of women.* (Working paper #2003-01). Boston, MA: Boston College Center for Retirement Research.

Meyers, J. (2001). *Age: 2000.* (Census 2000 Brief). Washington, D.C.: U.S. Census Bureau, C2KBR/01-12.

Morgan, D. L. (1998). Facts and figures about the baby boom. *Generations, 22*(1), 5-9.

National Academy on an Aging Society (2000, December). *Do young retirees and older workers differ by race?* (Data Profiles No. 4). Washington, D.C.: National Academy on an Aging Society, The Gerontological Society of America.

OWL (2002). *Social security privatization: A false promise for women.* (2002 Mother's Day Report). Washington, D.C.: Older Women's League.

Ozawa, M. N. & Law, S. W. (1992). Reported reasons for retirement: A study of recently retired workers. *Journal of Aging & Social Policy, 4*(3/4), 35-51.

Public Agenda Foundation (1997). *Miles to go: A status report on Americans.* New York: Public Agenda Foundation.

Quinn, J. F. (1999, February). *Retirement patterns and bridge jobs in the 1990s.* (EBRI Issue Brief). Washington, D.C.: Employee Benefit Research Institute.

Report of the Committee on Economic Security of 1935 (1985). (50th anniversary ed.). Washington, D.C.: National Conference on Social Welfare.

Retirement funds lose $1.5 billion due to Enron's fall. (2002, January 29). *The Oregonian*, C1.

Schulz, J. H. (2001). *The economics of aging.* (7th ed.). Westport, CN: Auburn House.

Schwab joins others ending contributions to 401(k)s. (2003, March 14). *New York Times*, C1.

Smeeding, T. M., Estes, C. L., & Glasse, L. (2000). *Social security in the 21st century.* (Issue Brief). Washington, D.C.: The Gerontological Society of America.

Social Security Act, 49 U.S.C. 620 (1935).

Social Security Act Amendments of 1939, 42 U.S.C. 403.

Social Security Administration, Office of Policy (2000). Fast facts and figures about social security. Washington, D.C.: U. S. Government Printing Office.

SPRY Foundation and National Committee to Preserve Social Security and Medicare (1999). *Redefining retirement: Research directions for America's diverse seniors.* Washington, D.C.: SPRY Foundation and National Committee to Preserve Social Security and Medicare.

Stanford, E. P. & Usita, P. M. (2002). Retirement: Who is at risk? *Generations, 26*(11), 45-48.

Texas Department of Aging (2000). *Texas baby boomer survey.* Austin, TX: Texas Department of Aging.

The 401(k) problem. (2002, December 1). *The Oregonian*, E1.

U.S. Bureau of the Census, (1998). *Measuring 50 years of economic change using the March Current Population Survey* (Current Population Reports P60-203). Washington, D.C.: U. S. Government Printing Office.

U.S. Census Bureau (1999). Married adults still in the majority. Retrieved January 7, 1999, from http://www.census.gov/Press-Releaseju/www.1999/cb99-03.html.

U.S. Census Bureau (2000). *Statistical abstract of the United States: 2000.* Washington, D.C.: U.S. Government Printing Office.

U.S. Census Bureau (2003). Economic briefing room. Retrieved March 26, 2003, from http://www.census.gov/cgi-bin/briefroom/BriefRm.

U.S. Department of Health and Human Services, Administration on Aging (2001). *Older women.* (Fact sheets from 2001 Older Americans Month). Retrieved April 6, 2002, from http://www.aoa.gov/may2000/FactSheets/OlderWomen.html.

U.S. Department of Labor, Employee Benefits Security Administration (2003). *Coverage status of workers under employer-provided pension plans.* Retrieved July 7, 2003, from http://www.dol.gov/ebsa.

U.S. Department of Labor, Pension and Welfare Benefits Administration (1993). *Trends in pensions.* Washington, D.C.: U. S. Government Printing Office.

Williamson, J. B. (1997). A critique of the case for privatizing social security. *The Gerontologist, 37*, 561-571.

Williamson, J. B. (2002). What's next for social security? Partial privatization? *Generations, 26*(11), 34-39.

Woods, J. R. (1994). Pension coverage among the baby boomers: Initial findings from a 1993 survey. *Social Security Bulletin, 57*(3), 12-25.

When Do Couples Expand Their ADL Caregiver Network Beyond the Marital Dyad?

Sheila Feld
Ruth E. Dunkle
Tracy Schroepfer

SUMMARY. Composition of caregiver networks (spouse only vs. others) for assistance with personal care limitations (ADLs) was examined in the AHEAD nationally representative sample of 215 elderly couples, using logistic regression. Findings showed network expansion beyond the spouse was influenced by a poor fit between solo spousal caregivers and caregiving tasks: Expanded networks were more likely when help recipi-

Sheila Feld is Professor Emerita of Social Work, The University of Michigan, School of Social Work, 1080 S. University, Ann Arbor, MI 48109-1106. Ruth E. Dunkle is Professor, The University of Michigan, School of Social Work, 1080 S. University, Ann Arbor, MI 48109-1106. Tracy Schroepfer is Assistant Professor of Social Work, University of Wisconsin-Madison, School of Social Work, 1350 University, Madison, WI 53706.

Address correspondence to: Sheila Feld, Professor Emerita of Social Work, The University of Michigan, School of Social Work, 1080 S. University, Ann Arbor, MI 48109-1106 (E-mail: sfeld@umich.edu).

An earlier version of this paper was presented at the Symposium on "Highlighting Interdependence in Mid Life and Late Life Married Couples" at the Annual Scientific Meeting of the Gerontological Society of America, Chicago, November 2001. Preparation of this paper was partially supported by NIA grant T32-AG00017.

[Haworth co-indexing entry note]: "When Do Couples Expand Their ADL Caregiver Network Beyond the Marital Dyad?" Feld, Sheila, Ruth E. Dunkle, and Tracy Schroepfer. Co-published simultaneously in *Marriage & Family Review* (The Haworth Press, Inc.) Vol. 37, No. 1/2, 2005, pp. 27-44; and: *Challenges of Aging on U.S. Families: Policy and Practice Implications* (ed: Richard K. Caputo) The Haworth Press, Inc., 2005, pp. 27-44. Single or multiple copies of this article are available for a fee from The Haworth Document Delivery Service [1-800-HAWORTH, 9:00 a.m. - 5:00 p.m. (EST). E-mail address: docdelivery@haworthpress.com].

ents had numerous health problems ($p < .01$) and ADL limitations ($p = .063$), and when spouses had any ADL limitations ($p < .01$). Expanded networks were also likely when couples included the wife as help recipient ($p < .05$), were Black ($p = .075$), and were in lengthy marriages ($p < .05$). Implications for theory, research, and family policy and practice are discussed. *[Article copies available for a fee from The Haworth Document Delivery Service: 1-800-HAWORTH. E-mail address: <docdelivery@haworthpress.com> Website: <http://www.HaworthPress.com> © 2005 by The Haworth Press, Inc. All rights reserved.]*

KEYWORDS. Spousal caregivers, ADL limitations, older couples, gender, marital duration

INTRODUCTION

Considerable evidence indicates that when a spouse is present, he or she is the predominant informal helper for community dwelling elders who need assistance with personal activities of daily living (ADLs) (Stone, Cafferata, & Sangl, 1987). Nevertheless, it is also clear that the spouse is not always the sole caregiver and that some spouses are not caregivers (Barrett & Lynch, 1999; Schulz, Newsom, Mittlemark, Burton, Hirsch, & Jackson, 1997). To date, however, only a few studies have investigated the circumstances under which elderly couples expand their caregiver network beyond the marital dyad to include help from other sources (Allen, 1994; Katz, Kabeto, & Langa, 2000; Stoller & Cutler, 1992) and only a limited number of such circumstances have been examined. More complete information on what circumstances influence couples to reach beyond each other, outside their usual care dyad, is important in order to design services for optimal care.

To redress this gap, it is essential that scholars expand the types of factors studied as influences on whether elderly couples rely solely on one another or include other helpers in their caregiver networks. Prior research has primarily addressed characteristics of care recipients that affect the spouse's role in the caregiver network (Allen, 1994; Katz et al., 2000; Stoller & Cutler, 1992). Although care recipients' assistance needs are clearly critical, further information is needed about which characteristics of the potential spouse caregivers and of couples as a unit might affect the expansion of caregiving networks beyond the spouse. One study has shown that potential spouse helpers who themselves have functional limitations are less likely to provide care to their partners (Katz et al., 2000). Research on how characteristics of informal caregivers affect the use of formal services has not focused on what particular characteristics of spouse caregivers influence their roles as caregivers (Bass & Noelker, 1987). Some studies of factors influencing sole reliance on the spousal caregiving assistance have examined a few characteristics of couples as a unit, such as gender, race, and availability of children (Allen, 1994; Stoller & Cutler, 1992). Other characteristics, though, such as the joint ages of couples and duration of their marriages were not investigated. Additionally, the available research has not always been based on representative samples of community-dwelling elders (Allen, 1994).

In this paper, we use a nationally representative sample to explore circumstances under which older married couples expand their Activities of Daily Living (ADL) caregiver networks beyond the spouse. We examine some key characteristics of care recipients, potential spouse helpers, and couples to identify those linked to networks composed solely of spouses and those linked to networks including other caregivers. The baseline sample of the Asset and Health Dynamics among the Oldest Old (AHEAD) survey (Soldo, Hurd, Rodgers, & Wallace, 1997) was used to identify caregiver networks among married elders 70 years of age and older. We focus on ADL networks because if such assistance is needed its receipt is essential to meet basic requirements of daily life. When caregiver networks are unable to provide adequate ADL aid, community-dwelling elders are often forced to enter nursing facilities (Aykan, 2002).

THEORETICAL PERSPECTIVES ON SPOUSAL CAREGIVING

Both Cantor's hierarchical compensatory models (Cantor & Brennan, 2000) and task-specific models (Litwak, 1985; Messeri, Silverstein, & Litwak, 1993) predict that spouses will be primary caregivers for their disabled partners, although for somewhat different reasons. In the hierarchical compensatory model, elders' preferences are the basis for care from persons in intimate personal rather than socially distant relationships. The task-specific model stresses the goodness of the match between characteristics of the marital dyad and specific personal caregiving tasks such as bathing and toileting (e.g., requirements for continually proximal and highly committed, but not technically skilled helpers). Unavailability of preferred intimate sources of help is critical to the hierarchical compensatory model's view of the circumstances under which other helpers provide care. Unfortunately, this model provides little guidance about why a co-resident spouse might not provide all necessary assistance. In the task-specific model, the time, energy, and skills required by caregiving tasks and the available time, energy, and skills of potential helpers are expected to affect the match between characteristics of caregiving tasks and potential helpers (Litwak, Jessop, & Moulton, 1994). The caregiving tasks for a partner in need of ADL assistance who has many ADL limitations, or who has numerous IADL limitations or multiple problematic health conditions, may require high levels of time, energy, or skills. Potential spouse helpers with functional limitations may have limited time, energy, or skills for caregiving. Either situation could result in poor matches between spouses and the provision of ADL care and could foster caregiver networks that include helpers other than the spouse.

Several strands of theory and research indicate that relying on one's marital partner for help is likely to be especially acceptable among couples who are older and/or in marriages of long duration. This work suggests that with increasing age and marital duration, partners are likely to exhibit high levels of interdependence and a more turning inward to the dyad for support. Although these ideas have not been linked specifically to the composition of caregiver networks, it seems reasonable to infer that greater interdependence may reduce the psychological acceptability of helpers outside the marital dyad. Carstensen and colleagues' socioemotional selectivity theory offers one possible explanation (Carstensen, Gottman, & Levenson, 1995; Carstensen, Isaacowitz, & Charles, 1999). They propose that as the perception of time left to live decreases with advanced age, elders selectively focus their social engagement on persons who enable them to maintain positive emotional states. The spouse is proposed to exemplify such a person, especially in long-term marriages. In such marriages, even when they are unhappy, older couples appear to have learned to regulate the expression of negative affect. Furthermore, a long history of reciprocal support and affirmation may allow frail elders to feel needed by the caregiving spouse and to avoid negative emotions linked to dependency. The help recipient may also be able to continue to provide emotional support to their spouse caregiver, thereby maintaining a sense of reciprocity. Alford-Cooper's (1998) study of couples married 50 years or more is consistent with these ideas. He reports that such couples exhibit high levels of interdependence based on long years of shared activities and experiences, regardless of the happiness of their marriage.

PRIOR EVIDENCE ON FACTORS AFFECTING THE COMPOSITION OF CAREGIVER NETWORK FOR MARRIED ELDERS

The limited available research is consistent with the task-specific model's suggestion that sole reliance on spousal help is more common when time, energy, and skills required by tasks are likely to match those of the spouse. Several studies show that when married help recipients have high levels of functional limitations, they are more likely to have non-spousal helpers (Miller & Guo, 2000; Mutchler & Bullers, 1994; Stoller & Cutler, 1992). Similarly, spouses' functional limitations decreased the likelihood that spouses provided care for the functional needs of their partners (Katz et al., 2000). In another study, spouses with serious health conditions were unlikely to provide care to their partners with functional limitations (Schulz & Beach, 1999).

Considerable evidence indicates that the receipt of spousal caregiving varies with the gender of the help recipient and caregiving spouse. Husbands are more likely to rely solely on their wives for support than wives are to rely solely on their husbands (Allen, 1994; Katz et al., 2000; Stoller & Cutler, 1992). The most common explanation for gender differences concerns societal female gender roles that include nurturance and caregiving. For elderly couples who accept this specialized gender role, wives are likely to have internalized the responsibility to care for their spouses and provided such care earlier in their marriage. Husbands are likely to expect care from their wives and to have less experience as a caregiver. It may, therefore, be more acceptable to both the caregiver and care recipient for the wife to provide all the needed care than for the husband to do so. Others outside the marital dyad may also be more likely to offer their supplemental support to a caregiving husband than to a caregiving wife.

Whether there are racial differences in reliance on spousal caregivers is unclear despite considerable research on racial differences in the acceptability of different types of caregivers. In the one identified study that addressed this issue in relation to sole reliance on spouses for either ADL or IADL assistance (Stoller & Cutler, 1992), Black and white elders did not differ. Most research with representative samples and multivariate controls has not found differences (Miller, Campbell, Davis, Furner, Giachello, Prohaska, Kaufman, Li, & Perez, 1996; Mutchler & Bullers, 1994). Yet, there is some evidence that the breadth of informal social support and caregiver networks is larger for Black than for white couples (Dilworth-Anderson & Burton, 1999; Stommel,

Given, & Given, 1998), but these studies did not focus on caregiving spouses. There is substantial evidence that, in general, availability of various potential caregivers affect the composition of elders' caregiver networks (Miller, McFall, & Campbell, 1994). Research on how availability of other informal and formal resources influences spousal caregiving is, however, limited and inconsistent. In one nationally representative study (Stoller & Cutler, 1992), elderly couples' numbers of sons and daughters or the presence of any proximate children did not affect sole reliance on spousal caregivers. Couples with very low or very high income were less likely to rely solely on spousal caregivers for ADL or IADL aid. Findings differed somewhat in a study of a convenience sample of married adults undergoing outpatient cancer treatment (Allen, Goldscheider, & Ciambrone, 1999). The presence of co-resident children reduced the likelihood that spouses were named as primary caregivers for assistance with functional needs, but number of other nearby children was not a significant factor.

Variables that might reflect the nature of the relationship between elderly couples have received little attention. This is surprising, given the assumption in both the hierarchical compensatory and task-specific models that reliance on the spouse for caregiving is based on high levels of intimacy and commitment. Other theories suggest also that couples who are older and in marriages of longer duration of marriage are more likely to rely primarily on one another. There is some evidence that the emotional ties between partners affect reliance on spousal caregiving. In their study of adults undergoing cancer treatment, Allen and colleagues (1999) found that the patient was more likely to name the spouse as the primary caregiver when the patient also identified the spouse as his/her emotional confidant. Spitze and Ward's (2000) study of a representative sample of middle-aged and older adults found that persons who described their marriage as happy were more likely to mention their spouse as someone who provided care when they were sick or needed personal care. Age of either care recipients or potential spouse helpers, but not both partners, has been investigated. Some studies found age was not tied to reliance on the spouse (Allen et al., 1999; Katz et al., 2000; Spitze & Ward, 2000), but in others older age was associated with less reliance on spousal caregiving (Mutchler & Bullers, 1994; Schulz et al., 1997). We did not locate any research examining reliance on spousal caregiving and the length of time couples have been married to one another. As marital duration might reflect the couples' commitment to one another and level of interdependence, it was included in the present study.

PRESENT STUDY

To extend prior research and theory, we used a representative sample to investigate the composition of ADL caregiver networks of elderly couples and focus on identifying those circumstances under which the spouse is the sole helper in the network and those under which networks include other helpers. We examined the effects of health and other characteristics of the help recipient member of a couple, functional impairment of the potential spouse helper member of the couple, and joint characteristics of the couple on network composition. The overall hypothesis was that sole reliance on the spouse for help with ADL limitations is less likely when the level of care required by the caregiving task does not match the ability of the spouse to provide that level of care, when other sources of help are readily available, or when other sources are psychologically acceptable to the couple.

METHODS

Sample

Data are from the first wave of the AHEAD survey, conducted in 1993-94 (see Soldo et al., 1997 for sampling details). This is a nationally representative sample of over 8,000 community-dwelling elders, aged 70 and older, and their spouses or partners.

The present paper was based on a subsample of the AHEAD respondents. The subsample included married couples (two co-residing persons who self-identified as spouses or partners) in which one partner was 70 years of age or older and received help with an ADL at least once a week. The ADLs were dressing, bathing, eating, toileting, walking across a room, and getting in or out of bed. A limitation was defined as the receipt of help or difficulty with any of these ADLs, or using equipment for walking or bed transfer. The subsample was restricted to recipients of help at least once a week because complete information on who provided help was obtained only in this circumstance. Additionally, the subsample was limited to couples where both members self-identified as Non-Hispanic white or as Non-Hispanic Black or African American because of evidence that race/ethnicity may affect network composition and the small number of couples in other racial/ethnic groups. The final subsample of 215 married couples resulted from these sample selection criteria and deletion of influential outliers identified by regression diagnostic procedures.

One member of each couple was designated the help recipient and the other the potential spouse helper. The help recipient was always a member of the couple who received ADL help at least weekly and was at least 70 years of age. In most of the 215 couples (80%, N = 147), only one partner met these criteria. In 47 couples, members met these criteria and one partner had more ADL limitations than the other one; for these couples, the partner with more limitations was designated the help recipient. For the one couple where both partners met these criteria and had equal numbers of ADL limitations, the help recipient was chosen at random.

Dependent Variable: ADL Caregiver Network

The dichotomous dependent variable distinguished couples with *Spouse Only* caregiver networks from those with *Other* caregiver networks. *Spouse Only* networks were those in which the only weekly help received with any of the six ADL limitations was from the spouse. *Other* caregiver networks were those in which any helper other than the spouse provided weekly assistance with one or more ADL limitation. The spouse could also have provided help, as was true for 41.9% of the couples with *Other* caregiver networks.

Predictor Variables

Characteristics of help recipients, spouses, and couples likely to affect ADL network composition were included as predictors. Three measures of poor health of help recipients were expected to be associated with increased caregiving demands on spouses and network expansion beyond the spouse. These were: (1) number of ADL limitations, as defined under sample selection criteria; (2) number of IADL limitations, defined as not being able to prepare a hot meal, shop for groceries, make a telephone call, or take medications without help or not doing the task because of health reasons; and (3) number of current health problems, including diabetes, heart condition, stroke, lung disease, cancer, arthritis, psychiatric problems, urine control, and legal blindness or very poor eyesight. Help recipients' Medicaid coverage was expected to affect availability of formal help and foster network expansion beyond the spouse.

Two aspects of the spouse's health were also expected to make the caregiving task more difficult for the spouse and to be associated with expansion of the caregiver network beyond the spouse. These were whether the spouse had any ADL limitations or IADL limitations.

Five characteristics of the couple that could influence the acceptability and/or availability of helpers other than the spouse were also used: gender of the help recipient and spouse; race (white/Black), number of proximate children; years married, and age. *Spouse Only* networks were expected to be more acceptable to couples with a male help recipient and female spouse than those with a female help recipient and male spouse. The expected effect of the couple's race was uncertain because of the inconsistencies in prior research noted previously (Dilworth-Anderson & Burton, 1999; Miller et al., 1996; Stoller & Cutler, 1992; Stommel et al., 1998). Availability of potential child helpers was expected to facilitate inclusion of helpers other than the spouse in caregiver networks, as measured by the couple's number of proximate children (those living less than 10 miles away, including co-residents). Some evidence suggested that longevity of a marriage and/or advanced age might foster sole reliance on the spouse (Alford-Cooper, 1998; Carstensen et al., 1999). To investigate these ideas, we used the number of years they had been married to one another and the sum of the couple's ages, as multicollinearity resulted if separate measures of the age of each of the partners were included.

Analytic Strategy

To handle the complex sample design, the Stata statistical package was used to obtain appropriate standard errors and significance levels. The weights used included adjustments for sample selection probabilities (clustering, over sampling of minority elders, and sampling both members of married couples), nonresponse, and deviations from the 1990 Census data.

A logistic regression model for categorical data was used to assess the independent impacts of the predictors on the composition of the ADL caregiver networks: *Spouse Only* networks were compared to the omitted referent category of *Other* networks. Odds ratios are reported to provide information on how variations in each predictor variable affected the odds of having a network consisting solely of the spouse. Significant odds ratios greater than 1.00 indicate the predictor increases the odds of *Spouse Only* networks; Odds ratios less than 1.00 indicate the predictor decreases the odds of *Spouse Only* networks (and increases the odds of *Other* networks). Because a one-unit change in odds for a continuous variable with a large range is often less meaningful than the odds associated with larger intervals (Hosmer, 2000), we report the odds ratio associated with 10 years of marriage. This odds ratio (and its associated confidence interval) was derived by exponentiating 10 times the beta for the Years Married variable.

RESULTS

Descriptive Findings

Table 1 shows that for most of these couples, as expected, regular help with ADL limitations came solely from within the couple (71.2%). Nevertheless, over a quarter of the couples (28.8%) had caregiver networks including helpers other than the spouse. Couples with *Other* caregiver networks included 12.1% in which there was at least one helper in addition to the spouse and 16.7% in which all help came from outside the marital dyad (data not shown).

The remainder of Table 1 shows the bivariate relationship between each predictor and network composition. *Spouse Only* networks were significantly more common when the help recipient had fewer ADL or IADL limitations and fewer problematic health conditions; the spouse had no ADL or IADL limitations; and the couple consisted of a male help recipient and female spouse, was white, was married relatively fewer years, and was younger. The help recipient's Medicaid coverage and the couple's number of proximate children were not significantly linked to network composition.

Multivariate Findings

The results of the logistic regression indicate the independent effects of each predictor variable on the composition of the ADL caregiver network are presented in Table 2. It shows that certain characteristics of the help recipient, the spouse, and the couple were significantly related to the composition of the caregiver networks.

ADL caregiver networks that included only the spouse were more common when the help recipient had relatively few ADL limitations ($p = .063$) and relatively few current health problems, but the number of IADLs did not significantly influence reliance on the spouse. Each additional ADL limitation of the help recipient reduced the odds of having

TABLE 1. Descriptive Differences Between Spouse Only and Other ADL Caregiver Networks

| Variable (Range) | ADL Network | | p |
| | Spouse Only | Other | |
	N = 153 (71.2%)	N = 62 (28.8%)	
Help Recipient Characteristics			
# of ADLs (1-6)	3.4	4.6	***
# of IADLs (0-4)	2.0	2.9	***
# of Conditions (0-5)	1.8	2.4	***
Medicaid			
No	94.1%	87.1%	
Yes	5.9%	12.9%	
Spouse Characteristics			
Any ADLs			***
No	83.0%	64.5%	
Yes	17.0%	35.5%	
Any IADLs			***
No	90.8%	71.0%	
Yes	9.2%	29.0%	
Couple Characteristics			
Gender			*
Female Recipient/Male Spouse	33.3%	64.5%	
Male Recipient/Female Spouse	66.7%	35.5%	
Race			*
White	86.3%	71.0%	
Black	13.7%	29.0%	
# Proximate Children (0-6)	1.0	1.2	
Sum of Partners' Ages (128-187)	153.7	157.6	**
Years Married (1-76)	47.1	52.4	**

Note. Entries are means unless noted otherwise. Means and percentages are based on raw data. All significance tests take design effects into account by using the Stata software.
$*p \le .05$ $**p \le .01$ $***p \le .001$

a *Spouse Only* network by 26% and each additional current health problem reduced these odds by 30%.

Spouse Only networks were also more common if the spouse had no ADL limitations, but whether or not the spouse had IADL limitations did not significantly influence network composition. Spouses with

TABLE 2. Logistic Regression Model for Spouse Only Compared to Other ADL Caregiver Networks (N = 215)

Variable	Odds Ratio	Confidence Interval
Help Recipient Characteristics		
# of ADLs	0.74+	(0.54, 1.02)
# of IADLs	0.76	(0.49, 1.18)
# of Conditions	0.70**	(0.54, 0.90)
Medicaid (No/Yes)	0.76	(0.24, 2.44)
Spouse Characteristics		
Any ADLs (No/Yes)	0.30**	(0.12, 0.73)
Any IADLs (No/Yes)	0.98	(0.39, 2.43)
Couple Characteristics		
Gender (Female Recipient/Male Recipient)	3.42*	(1.20, 9.72)
Race (White/Black)	0.37+	(0.12, 1.11)
# Proximate Children	1.04	(0.71, 1.55)
Sum of Partners' Ages	0.98	(0.94, 1.02)
Years Married[a]	0.76*	(0.68, 0.80)

Note. The overall model was significant, p = .002.
[a]Odds ratio and confidence interval based on 10-year intervals.
$+p \leq .10$ $*p \leq .05$ $**p \leq .01$.

ADL limitations were 70% less likely than those without ADL limitations to be the sole caregivers for their partners.

Some of the couple's joint characteristics also affected sole reliance on spousal help. *Spouse Only* networks were more common when the couple included a male help recipient and female spouse, was white ($p = .075$), or had been married to each other for relatively few years, but the couple's ages and number of proximate children did not have significant effects. Male help recipients were over three times more likely to rely solely on their wives for care than female help recipients were to receive care only from their husbands. Black couples were 63% less likely than white ones to have networks consisting only of the spouse. The direction of the effect for marital duration was unexpected: for each 10 years the couple had been married, the odds of sole reliance on the spouse for caregiving was reduced by 24%.

DISCUSSION

Present findings reinforce other evidence that spouses do not always provide all the care received by their elderly disabled partners. In this nationally representative sample of Black and white elders and their spouses/partners, over a quarter of the elders received regular assistance with personal care limitations from someone other than their spouse; nearly 17% received no assistance from their spouse. Similar figures were reported by Schulz et al. (1997), in a representative sample of married persons 65 years and older drawn from four geographic areas. Overall, 19% of those elders who had any ADL or IADL limitation received no help from their spouse. These findings demonstrate the importance of policy and program designers understanding the circumstances under which spouses provide care. The present study contributes to this issue by identifying not only characteristics of help recipients that affect spousal caregiving, but also those of potential spouse helpers and couples as a unit.

Based on the task-specific model and prior empirical evidence, we proposed several circumstances under which caregiver networks would be likely to expand beyond the spouse because of a poor fit between the time, energy, or skills of solo spouse caregivers and of the required personal care tasks. Several of the multivariate results supported these expectations. Networks that included helpers other than the spouse were more common when the help recipient had a relatively high number of problematic health conditions and the spouse had any personal care needs; the help recipient's number of personal care limitations tended to show a similar effect. Some prior research has also shown that greater health difficulties of the help recipient or the spouse lessen reliance on spousal caregivers (Allen et al., 1999; Katz et al., 2000; Schulz et al., 1997, 1999; Stoller & Cutler, 1992). The present study appears to be the only one based on a representative sample of elders that has examined the simultaneous effects of the health of both partners on solo spousal caregiving in multivariate analyses. Whereas the descriptive findings indicated that help recipients and spouses in ADL networks that included caregivers beyond the spouse had significantly more IADL limitations, this was not the case when other factors were considered. This suggests that other co-existing health difficulties, such as ADL limitations and chronic health problems, have stronger independent effects on ADL caregiver network composition than do IADL limitations.

We also expected that the availability of other potential sources of help would foster expansion of the caregiver network beyond the spouse. However, neither the help recipient's Medicaid coverage nor the couple's number of proximate children was significant in the descriptive or multivariate findings. The lack of effect for availability of children is consistent with Stoller and Cutler's (1992) study of elders' sole reliance on spousal ADL or IADL caregivers. One reason for these negative findings may be that Medicaid facilitates expansion to include formal caregivers and proximate children facilitate network expansion to include adult child caregivers. The relatively small number of couples with networks that included any helper other than the spouse meant that we were unable to analyze separately these different types of expanded networks. Studies with larger samples are needed to investigate the impact of these and other availability measures on various types of caregiver networks that extend beyond the spouse. Another possibility worth pursuing is that characteristics of adult children other than their geographic proximity are relevant to their inclusion in caregiver networks, such as their own health problems, marital status, gender, beliefs in filial responsibility, or emotional ties to their parents. The impact of other potential sources of informal support such as other relatives and friends on extension of caregiver networks beyond the spouse also warrants attention.

Certain characteristics of the couple as a unit were also predicted to be associated with network expansion beyond the spouse because they were expected to influence preferences for help from the spouse and the acceptability of help received from caregivers other than the spouse. The findings confirm some of these predictions. As expected, when the help recipient was female and the spouse was male, caregiver networks were more likely to include helpers other than the spouse than to consist solely of the spouse. This finding confirms considerable prior research on gender differences in spousal caregiving (e.g., Allen, 1994; Stoller & Cutler, 1992) and is one of the few studies that also indicates the importance of gender even when health of both partners is taken into account (Katz et al., 2000).

Race had a marginally significant effect. Black couples were more likely than white ones to have networks that included helpers outside the marital dyad, which is consistent with some prior studies, but not others. But the comparison is difficult to make, as we are aware of no prior research on this topic that has controlled for spouse's health, which is likely to be worse for Black than for white couples.

The present study appears to be the first one to test the idea that elderly couples in marriages of long duration and/or those at advanced ages would be prone to rely on spousal caregiving for help with personal care needs, as suggested by theories of socio-emotional selectivity and interdependence (Alford-Cooper, 1998; Carstensen et al., 1999). Our findings were contrary to this expectation. At the bivariate level, couples whose caregiver networks consisted solely of the spouse were in marriages of shorter durations and were younger than those whose networks extended beyond the spouse. These differences might have reflected the better health of younger couples. The multivariate findings helped us evaluate this possibility and determine if the couple's ages as well as the longevity of their marriage were important when considered simultaneously. Only marital duration remained significant: the longer a couple had been married to one another, the less likely it was that the spouse would provide all the ADL care received by the disabled partner and the more likely it was that the caregiver network would include help from outside the marital dyad.

How aid from outside the marital dyad affects a couple's sense of personal control over their life together may help us understand these findings about marital longevity. The social support and caregiving literature has addressed this issue from the perspective of the threats to independence that help recipients and caregivers may experience when getting support (e.g., Krause, 1990; O'Connor, 1995). However, it does not appear to have explored what it might mean for an elderly couple to acknowledge they can no longer independently carry out what they and most of society probably assume is their mutual responsibility of caring for one another. The present findings may indicate that elderly couples in longer and shorter marriages differ in the subjective meaning they place on getting help from outside the dyad. Couples in lengthy marriages may develop a convoy of social supporters with a long history of reciprocal aid. This history may enable the couple to draw on this support bank for caregiving without feeling overly dependent (Antonucci & Jackson, 1990). Marital longevity may also engender a strong sense of integrity as a marital unit. This could mean that accepting help from outside the dyad is less likely to arouse threats to the couple's sense of independence and the negative emotions that can accompany such threats. Future research could address these possibilities by exploring the reasons couples give for continuing to rely only on one another for help even when other sources of help may be available. This information could be valuable to practitioners and program designers who frequently face situations in which elderly couples resist accepting help from outside the marital dyad even when the caregiver is under considerable stress (O'Connor). Unfortunately, the AHEAD survey and other large representative studies of the elderly do not provide the kinds of data necessary to address these issues.

At present, the reasons for the findings about the couple's marital duration are uncertain. Nonetheless, they show the value of understanding how characteristics of the couple as a unit affect their caregiver network composition. The importance of viewing the couple as a unit is also seen in the findings that aspects of the health of both the help recipient and the spouse were important determinants of the locus of help received. These findings support Schulz and Beach's (1999) recommendation that health practitioners assess a couple's health, not just that of the identified patient, to determine the couple's need for assistance from outside the marital dyad. This assessment may also help identify couples who would be willing to accept such help.

Despite these contributions, we recognize several limitations in the study. The cross-sectional nature of the design prevents firm conclusions about the causal direction of some of the associations. This design also does not illuminate the dynamic ways in which changes in the health of members of the marital dyad and changes in caregiver network composition are inter-related. Because of the relatively small number of couples whose networks included helpers other than the spouse, we were unable to consider who these other helpers were or to investigate whether the same or different circumstances are associated with networks that include formal helpers and that include specific types of informal helpers other than the spouse. The required restriction of the sample to those with ADL limitations who received assistance at least once a week meant that the role of spousal caregivers remains unclear for elders who receive no help or infrequent help, and who may have unmet ADL needs.

Nevertheless, we believe that the present findings highlight the importance of researchers, policy makers, and practitioners recognizing that older marital couples do not always rely solely on one another for assistance with personal care limitations. In addition, familiarity by these professionals with the circumstances under which caregiver network expansion is likely could be useful. Family practitioners who are assessing the need for outside assistance in elderly married couples may find it valuable to consider the needs and desires of the couple as a unit. Identification of couples in which both members of the pair have personal care limitations is important, as they may be most in need of additional caregiving resources and most willing to accept them. The gender and race of both members of the couple, as well as the longevity of their relationship, may also be important aspects of the couple's willingness or resistance to accepting assistance from outside the dyad. Finally, an assessment of the subjective meaning a couple places on outside assistance may help practitioners understand the couple's readiness and reluctance for such help.

NOTE

1. Years married was based on the report of the help recipient, except that the report of the spouse was used when there was no report from the help recipient, or when the reports of the help recipient and spouse differed by five or more years and the help recipient had severe cognitive problems and the spouse did not.

REFERENCES

Alford-Cooper, F. (1998). *For keeps: Marriages that last a lifetime.* Armonk, NY: M. E. Sharpe.

Allen, S. M. (1994). Gender differences in spousal caregiving and unmet need for care. *Journal of Gerontology: Social Sciences, 49,* S187-195.

Allen, S. M., Goldscheider, F., & Ciambrone, D. A. (1999). Gender roles, marital intimacy, and nomination of spouse as primary caregiver. *The Gerontologist, 39,* 150-158.

Antonucci, T. C. & Jackson, J. S. (1990). The role of reciprocity in social support. In I.G. Sarason, B. R. Sarason, & G. R. Pierce (Eds.), *Social support: An interactional view* (pp. 173-198). New York: Wiley.

Aykan, H. (2002). Do state Medicaid policies affect the risk of nursing home entry among the elderly? Evidence from the AHEAD study. *Research on Aging, 24,* 487-512.

Barrett, M. E. & Lynch, S. M. (1999). Caregiving networks of elderly persons: Variation by marital status. *The Gerontologist, 39,* 695-704.

Bass, D. & Noelker, L. (1987). The influence of family caregivers on elders' use of in-home services. *Journal of Health and Social Behavior, 28,* 184-196.

Cantor, M. H. & Brennan, M. (2000). *Social care of the elderly: The effects of ethnicity, class, and culture.* New York: Springer.

Carstensen, L. L., Gottman, J. M., & Levenson, R. W. (1995). Emotional behavior in long-term marriage. *Psychology and Aging, 10,* 140-149.

Carstensen, L. L., Isaacowitz, D. M., & Charles, S. T. (1999). Taking time seriously: A theory of socioemotional selectivity. *American Psychologist, 54,* 165-181.

Dilworth-Anderson, P. & Burton, L. (1999). Critical issues in understanding family support and older minorities. In T. P. Miles (Ed.), *Full color aging* (pp. 93-105). Washington, DC: Gerontological Society of America.

Hosmer, D. W. (2000). *Applied logistic regression* (2nd ed.). New York: Wiley.

Katz, St. J., Kabeto, M., & Langa, K. M. (2000). Gender disparities in the receipt of home care for elderly people with disability in the United States. *Journal of the American Medical Association, 284,* 3022-3027.

Krause, N. (1990). Stress, social support, and well-being in later life: Focusing on salient social roles. In M. A. P. Stephens, J. H. Crowther, S. E. Hobfoll, & D. L.

Tennenbaum (Eds.), *Stress and coping in later life families* (pp. 71-97). New York: Hemisphere Publishing.

Litwak, E. (1985). *Helping the elderly: The complementary roles of informal networks and formal systems*. New York: Guilford Press.

Litwak, E., Jessop, D. J., & Moulton, H. J. (1994). Optimal use of formal and informal systems over the life course. In E. Kahana, D. E. Biegel, & M. L. Wykle (Eds.), *Family caregiving across the lifespan* (pp. 96-132). Thousand Oaks, CA: Sage.

Messeri, P., Silverstein, M., & Litwak, E. (1993). Choosing optimal support groups: A review and reformulation. *Journal of Health and Social Behavior, 34*, 122-137.

Miller, B., Campbell, R. T., Davis, L., Furner, S., Giachello, A., Prohaska, T., Kaufman, J. E., Li, M., & Perez, C. (1996). Minority use of community long-term care services: A comparative analysis. *Journal of Gerontology: Social Sciences, 51B*, S70-S81.

Miller, B. & Guo, S. (2000). Social support for spouse caregivers of persons with dementia. *Journal of Gerontology: Social Sciences, 55B*, S163-172.

Miller, B., McFall, S., & Campbell, R. T. (1994). Changes in sources of community long-term care among African American and white frail older persons. *Journal of Gerontology: Social Sciences, 49*, S14-24.

Mutchler, J. E. & Bullers, S. (1994). Gender differences in formal care use in later life. *Research on Aging, 16*, 235-250.

O'Connor, D. L. (1995).Caring for a memory-impaired spouse: A gender-sensitive perspective. *Journal of Women & Aging, 7*, 24-42.

Schulz, R. & Beach, S. R. (1999). Caregiving as a risk factor for mortality: The caregiver health effects study. *Journal of the American Medical Association, 282*, 215-219.

Schulz, R., Newsom, J., Mittlemark, M., Burton, L., Hirsch, C., & Jackson, S. (1997). Health effects of caregiving: The caregiver health effects study: An ancillary study of "The Cardiovascular Health Study." *Annals of Behavioral Medicine, 19*, 110-116.

Soldo, B. J., Hurd, M. D., Rodgers, W. L., & Wallace, R. B. (1997). Asset and health dynamics among the oldest old: An overview of the AHEAD study. *Journal of Gerontology, Series B, 52B (Special Issue)*, 1-20.

Spitze, G. & Ward, R. (2000). Gender, marriage, and expectations for personal care. *Research on Aging, 22*, 451-469.

Stoller, E. P. & Cutler, S. J. (1992). The impact of gender on configurations of care among elderly couples. *Research on Aging, 14*, 313-330.

Stommel, M., Given, C. W., & Given, B. A. (1998). Racial differences in the division of labor between primary and secondary caregivers. *Research on Aging, 20*, 199-217.

Stone, R., Cafferata, G. L., & Sangl, J. (1987). Caregivers of the frail elderly: A national profile. *The Gerontologist, 27*, 616-626.

Family-Based Intervention
in Residential Long-Term Care

Joseph E. Gaugler
Keith A. Anderson
Heidi H. Holmes

SUMMARY. Family care for older adults is often conceptualized as a 'career,' and one of the key transitions that may occur during the course of caregiving is the placement of an older relative in a residential long-term care facility (most commonly a nursing home). This literature review critiques and synthesizes existing intervention strategies designed to promote family involvement following institutionalization. In particular, two types of family-based interventions are identified that have received scientific evaluations in the literature: group-based and family-staff partnership approaches. Specific studies on each of these types ($N = 11$) are summarized and critiqued. Key research and practice recommendations are

Joseph E. Gaugler is Assistant Professor, Department of Behavioral Science, The University of Kentucky, 110 College of Medicine Office Building, Lexington, KY 40536-0086. Keith A. Anderson is Research Assistant, PhD Program in Gerontology, The University of Kentucky, 110 College of Medicine Office Building, Lexington, KY 40536-0086. Heidi H. Holmes is Research Assistant, PhD Program in Gerontology, The University of Kentucky, 110 College of Medicine Office Building, Lexington, KY 40536-0086.

Address correspondence to: Joseph E. Gaugler, Assistant Professor, Department of Behavioral Science, The University of Kentucky, 110 College of Medicine Office Building, Lexington, KY 40536-0086 (E-mail: jgaugle@uky.edu).

[Haworth co-indexing entry note]: "Family-Based Intervention in Residential Long-Term Care." Gaugler, Joseph E., Keith A. Anderson, and Heidi H. Holmes. Co-published simultaneously in *Marriage & Family Review* (The Haworth Press, Inc.) Vol. 37, No. 1/2, 2005, pp. 45-62; and: *Challenges of Aging on U.S. Families: Policy and Practice Implications* (ed: Richard K. Caputo) The Haworth Press, Inc., 2005, pp. 45-62. Single or multiple copies of this article are available for a fee from The Haworth Document Delivery Service [1-800-HAWORTH, 9:00 a.m. - 5:00 p.m. (EST). E-mail address: docdelivery@haworthpress.com].

http://www.haworthpress.com/web/MFR
Digital Object Identifier: 10.1300/J002v37n01_05

also offered to guide the future evaluation of programs to assist families adapt to the long-term care experience. *[Article copies available for a fee from The Haworth Document Delivery Service: 1-800-HAWORTH. E-mail address: <docdelivery@ haworthpress.com> Website: <http://www.HaworthPress.com> © 2005 by The Haworth Press, Inc. All rights reserved.]*

KEYWORDS. Family involvement, family caregiving

INTRODUCTION

Families have long been considered the key providers of intensive long-term care to disabled, community-based older people in the U.S. (Whitlatch & Noelker, 1996). However, studies on life and quality of life in the nursing home have taken note of how family involvement following institutionalization may account for positive outcomes on the part of residents, family members, and even staff (Kiely, Simon, Jones, & Morris, 2000; Penrod, Kane, & Kane, 2000). In particular, a series of interventions have been evaluated to assist caregiving families remain effectively involved in the lives of loved ones well after institutionalization. Despite the emergence of a number of programmatic approaches to help families adapt to the nursing home transition, no efforts to date have attempted to critically integrate existing findings.

The goal of this research review is to summarize and critique research on family-based intervention in residential long-term care. Following the review of strategies designed to enhance family integration in the nursing home, a series of research and practice recommendations are forwarded to guide the design, implementation, and evaluation of future interventions. We anticipate this review will serve as a key resource for researchers and practitioners interested in facilitating families' transition to the nursing home experience.

METHODS

A multi-component strategy was implemented to identify evaluations of family-based interventions in residential long-term care. We initially conducted an extensive search on the MEDLINE, PSYCINFO, and CINAHL databases, mapping onto the following subject headings: 'family involvement in long-term care,' 'families in nursing homes,' 'interventions in nursing homes,' 'delay of nursing home placement,' and 'delay of institutionalization.' References identified from this search of the literature and published between 1970 and 2003 were examined for potential inclusion. Dissertation abstracts were excluded. A snowball approach was also used where the references of studies located in our initial database searches were examined to identify additional analyses of interest. Finally, secondary searches of the MEDLINE, PSYCINFO, and CINAHL databases of prominent authors in the family involvement literature (e.g., Maas, Pillemer) offered other potential studies for review. Given the widespread, multidisciplinary review conducted, studies hailed from journals ranging from gerontology and family relations (e.g., *The Gerontologist*; *Family Systems*), to social work (e.g., *Journal of Gerontological Social Work*) to nursing (e.g., *Journal of Gerontological Nursing*).

Selected articles met the following criteria: (1) interventions focused on or included family members of older adults in nursing homes or similar residential care settings; and (2) an attempt was made by investigators to systematically evaluate outcomes from the family-based program (e.g., satisfaction, family involvement, resident outcomes, etc.). Studies that simply described existing programs but did not conduct an evaluation were excluded in the final review. The initial search of the literature yielded over 100 studies dealing with family involvement in nursing homes and long-term care. After the application of our review criteria, 21 studies were identified that described family-based interventions in residential long-term care, and of these 11 were subject to any type of evaluation. The latter group of evaluations served as the source of the current literature review. We then organized the review by identifying whether commonalities existed in the types of programs evaluated, and two main intervention types were found: group-based approaches (e.g., family support groups, family councils) and family-staff partnership/care planning approaches. Interventions are summarized and critiqued by type for the purposes of the subsequent literature review.

RESULTS

Various interventions have attempted to facilitate family involvement and improve quality of staff-family relationships. Although a number of strategies have been proposed and described in the literature, including support groups, family councils, solution-based therapies, and family-staff conflict resolution, most studies describe rather than evaluate family-based interventions (e.g., Cox & Ephross, 1989; Fabisewski & Howell, 1986; Greenfield, 1984; Hansen, Patterson, & Wilson, 1988; Numerof, 1983; Sancier, 1984; Shulman & Mandel, 1988; Sidell, 1997; Van Meter & Johnson, 1985; Vinton, Mazza, & Kim, 1998). Programs that were subject to evaluation are discussed below.

Group Approaches

Early research on support groups and family volunteer programs generally utilized non-scientific designs and small samples to evaluate their respective interventions. For example, periodic support groups developed by Safford (1980) and Helphand and Porter (1982) as well as a 'family council' initiated by Palmer (1991) tended to include small numbers of family members (10-20). Each of these approaches had as their objectives to assist family members find an appropriate role in caring for and interacting with residents in the nursing home (NH), offer support to family members when adjusting to NH care, and in some cases (Palmer, 1991) include administration and staff to address family concerns. Open-ended questionnaires administered at the conclusion of each of these programs indicated that family members were satisfied with participation. However, other important outcomes (e.g., family involvement, staff-resident relationships) were not rigorously evaluated.

Subsequent group approaches implemented more complex strategies when attempting to facilitate family involvement following relatives' institutionalization. For example, Linsk and colleagues (Linsk, Miller, Pflaum, & Ortigara-Vick, 1988) developed and evaluated a program that included family-staff meetings and family education courses for 45 family members of Alzheimer's patients and staff. The goal of the intervention was to establish a clear delineation of responsibilities and a sense of partnership between participating family members and staff and increase family involvement. Over a nine-month period, 25 family members who completed follow-up interviews indicated that they felt closer to their relatives. A family support program developed by Marsden (1990) had as its primary objectives to increase the knowledge of NH facilities' services and care responsibilities and help families become more comfortable in the NH setting. A parallel education and training program was also administered to improve staff members' interaction and communication with residents. Of the 242 individuals who responded to a post-evaluation mail survey (number of family or staff were not specified), 76% reported they learned "very much." Participants also reported a number of behavior changes, such as improved quality of visits and interaction with NH residents and increased provision of socioemotional support. A more recent intervention implemented an educational support program for family members of newly-admitted NH residents (Peak, 2000) with the objective of helping family members take greater enjoyment in visiting relatives as well as improving family attitudes toward staff. The educational-support program included group sessions that were held three times over a 15-month time period; these sessions provided participants with the opportunity to share experiences of placement, exchange information, and tips on adaptation following a loved one's institutionalization, and, with the help of a social worker, identify activities that would improve family visits. In addition to improving family members' attitudes, the number of family members who reported enjoyment of their visits to the NH doubled by the end of the program. These evaluations suggest the potential of family orientation approaches to facilitate involvement over time. However, the limited samples of residents and facilities attenuate the findings. Some of the studies used post-test designs only, making it difficult to determine the actual impact of the program on family member attitudes or behaviors. In addition, control groups may have provided more insight into the effectiveness of these programs.

The National Citizens' Coalition for Nursing Home Reform (NCCNHR, 1998) conducted a national survey of long-term care ombudsman in each state of the U.S. to determine how advocates successfully involve families in NH care. A total of 106 questionnaires were completed (the 52 state ombudsmen were asked to forward surveys to other key regional advocates in their particular states). The open-ended data compiled suggested that family councils provided participants with a united, credible voice in NH care, helped to integrate and facilitate ombudsman efforts in advocating for the rights of residents, and challenged NHs to provide improved care by identifying important problems in the facility and raising such issues to staff and administration. Barriers identified in the national report included facility resistance to hinder family council meetings and advocacy efforts (e.g., inappropriate meeting locations, insisting that staff attend), the potential of council meetings to become 'gripe' sessions, difficulties in organizing and recruiting family members with hectic lifestyles, and leadership issues. While the NCCNHR report offers a tremendous resource for how family councils can be effectively implemented in NHs, findings were based largely on advocates' post hoc perspectives (some of whom were family members of NH residents at the time of the report or before and others who were not). A determination of whether family councils operate to effectively improve family, resident, or staff outcomes was not addressed through a prospective evaluation design that included family, resident, and/or staff assessments.

Family-Staff Approaches

Other efforts have focused on having individual family members and staff meet to discuss care responsibilities, develop methods to alleviate concerns, and improve the nature of family visits and involvement. For example, a smaller-scale but rigorous study by Anderson, Hobson, Steiner, and Rodel (1992) ascertained whether family collaboration in the development of care plans would exert positive benefits on NH residents suffering from dementia and improve family attitudes toward visits and involvement. Six family members were randomized to an experimental condition, where two registered nurses met with family members to design and develop care plans, identify resident interests, and address care concerns collaboratively. The remaining six family members were randomized to a usual care control. Three months later, nurses and family members in the treatment group met to evaluate their collaborative care plan experience. Post-test measures found that family members in the experimental condition reported significantly better relations with the resident and indicated that the resident responded more favorably to family visits. Also, medications were more likely to be reduced for residents in the experimental condition. The findings emphasize the potential benefits of implementing flexible, family-staff partnership interventions to facilitate communication and effectively address the concern of each family member. A particular strength of this study was including a control group as part of its experimental design, which helped to highlight the benefits of the program. However, replications with larger samples are needed to better discern the actual benefits for families, staff, and residents.

Qualitative research by Hepburn and colleagues (Caron, Hepburn, Luptak, Grant, Ostwald, & Keenan, 1999; Hepburn, Caron, Luptak, Ostwald, Grant, & Keenan, 1997) examined the use of reminiscence and narratives in improving family and resident adaptation to the NH context. The 'Family Stories' approach consists of six to eight family group sessions that include multiple family members and are held over a two-month period. Family members are encouraged by project staff to complete exercises designed to create a narrative of the institutionalized relative's life. These biographies are later presented to staff to help personalize the resident and provide NH staff with more intimate knowledge of residents' interests, histories, and families. Initial open-ended analysis suggested that families had stronger social connections than more traditional programs (e.g., family councils or support groups) and avoided discussing disease-related aspects of residents in favor of personalizing the resident's life in the facility. The program developed by Hepburn and associates is a potentially innovative approach to improving staff-family-resident relations in the NH context. However, more extensive empirical evaluations of the Biography Project that demonstrate the impact of this program on family involvement and resident outcomes would further emphasize the roles of families in transforming traditional approaches to NH care.

The larger-scale Family Involvement in Care (FIC) program was specifically designed to negotiate and establish partnerships and roles between NH staff (e.g., nurse's aides) and family members of cognitively impaired residents (Maas, Swansom, Buckwalter, Lenth, & Specht, 2000). The FIC consisted of multiple components that combined the group approaches described above with specific activities to enhance family-staff partnerships. Program components included family orientation and education sessions as well as sessions between individual family members and staff to negotiate and evaluate care responsibilities. The goal of the intervention was to improve family members' involvement and adaptation to placement, enhance staff members' perceptions of family members, and improve staff job satisfaction. The FIC was evaluated in 14 NH special care units (7 experimental, 7 control) for Alzheimer's residents in Iowa. Since randomization was not possible, experimental and control facilities were matched on important characteristics (e.g., size). A nine-month trial of the FIC was completed for each family member. Staff members were measured at baseline and every 6 months thereafter. Two hundred family members agreed to be contacted of the 371 that signed consent forms, and 99 family members completed follow-up interviews during the nine-month evaluation period. Following participation in the FIC, family members provided more physical care and their consideration of the personal needs of the resident increased. Moreover, feelings of loss decreased for family members in the FIC. Strength of partnership ratings between family members and staff were also higher in the FIC. The FIC evaluation demonstrates the potential benefits of structured interventions for improving family involvement. However, the study also illustrates the challenges facing researchers who attempt to evaluate similar interventions; refusals and attrition were especially high among family members, and the lack of a true randomized design may have biased the final empirical results.

Pillemer, Suiter, Henderson, Meador, Schulz, Robison, and Hegeman (2003) developed a similar multicomponent approach. The Partners in Caregiving (PIC) program was designed to assist family members through councils and support groups and collaborations with staff and administrators to create a more family-oriented facility environment. Two workshop series (one for nurses and nursing assistants; one for family members) included training in communication and listening skills, group discussions, and similar exercises. Objectives of the PIC were to improve family involvement in NHs, facilitate relationships between families and staff, and enhance staff job satisfaction. Evaluation of the PIC included 932 relatives and 655 staff members recruited from 20 NHs in the state of New York (Pillemer et al., 2003). Two representative units from ten of the facilities were randomly assigned to a treatment or control condition, and participants (family members, residents, and staff) were recruited from these units. Ten additional facilities were randomly selected as 'pure' control sites to reduce the potential effects of contamination. After six months, 683 family members and 450 staff completed follow-up interviews (interviews were administered at baseline, two months, and six months). Significant results were found over the two- and six-month intervals; both families and staff in the PIC showed improved attitudes toward each other, family members reported decreased conflict with staff, and staff were less likely to quit during the six-month course of the intervention. The findings suggest that the PIC may serve as an effective method to reduce family-staff conflict in NHs. However, several limitations may attenuate these conclusions. Treatment effects appeared to weaken from the 2- to 6-month time interval. The authors also suggest that more intensive tracking of policy and procedural changes within facilities must be completed to gain a better understanding of how family-staff interventions can change the environment of NHs.

Methodological and Conceptual Limitations of Family-Based Interventions

A number of approaches have been proposed to help family members remain engaged in the lives of their loved ones in NHs. However, there remain few rigorous evaluations that demonstrate the overall efficacy of such interventions. Most evaluations are more intent on describing programs than actually evaluating them. Small sample sizes and short-term evaluation periods (often due to attrition in recruited samples) pose particular empirical challenges that require more advanced statistical and design approaches. As prior research has shown, while many residents who are admitted to a NH die soon thereafter (up to 24% following the first three months after placement (see Aneshensel, Pearlin, Mullan, Zarit, & Whitlatch, 1995), additional work has demonstrated that increased family involvement, ranging from visits to socioemotional support to ADL care, is strongly associated with decreased mortality and/or increased discharge among NH samples (Kiely et al., 2000; Penrod et al., 2000). These findings suggest the wide range of benefits family involvement may provide. However, measured outcomes often do not extend far beyond participant satisfaction; indicators such as family involvement, resident quality of life, quality of care, or resident mortality are often not considered.

In addition to issues in design and evaluation, another limitation in family-based interventions is the sole focus on one 'primary' family member. Given that multiple family members may be involved in the care of a loved one in a residential facility and vary in their relationship to the resident, programs are likely to exert the greatest benefits if they take the complexity of family structure into account in their particular protocols. Similarly, existing family-involvement interventions include predominately Caucasian samples; given the differences in care provision, cultural meanings, and perceptions ascribed to caregivers of various ethnic and racial backgrounds, it is necessary to determine whether the approaches described above are flexible enough to meet the needs of diverse families. Many of the existing family-based intervention programs are also atheoretical; there appears to be a lack of conceptual or theoretical models designed to specify the processes leading to increased family involvement and improved outcomes in each of these programs. Finally, few approaches are targeted to families dealing with newly admitted NH residents and the challenges of navigating the long-term care experience.

RECOMMENDATIONS

Research Recommendations

Conceptualization of family care. A limitation of family-based intervention research is its general focus on a 'primary' family member. The primary family member generally refers to the one relative who remains most involved in the life of a resident following institutionalization (Maas et al., 2000). As the community-based caregiving literature has noted, there is usually one 'primary' caregiver who provides the bulk of assistance to a disabled elderly relative (Aneshensel et al., 1995; Cantor, 1983). However, other studies have emphasized that multiple family members within diverse family structures provide assistance to chronically impaired older adults, illustrating the complexity of the family caregiving process (Dilworth-Anderson, 2001; Schoenberg, Amey, Stoller, & Mundoon, in press; Tennstedt, McKinlay, & Sullivan, 1989), and that including multiple family members in psychoeducational interventions is likely to exert the most positive impact on care recipient outcomes (e.g., Mittelman, Epstein, & Pierzchala, 2003). In addition, as descriptive caregiving research has consistently emphasized, kin relationship to the older care recipient is a key indicator of type of assistance provided (e.g., spouses tend to provide more intensive, hands-on, ADL type of care; see Stone, Cafferata, & Stangl, 1987; Tennstedt, McKinlsy, & Sullivan, 1993), time to institutionalization (adult children are more likely to institutionalize sooner; see Gaugler, Kane, Kane, Clay, & Newcomer, 2003), and is also predictive of greater family conflict and depression following placement in a nursing home (Gaugler, Zarit, & Pearlin, 1999; Grau, Teresi, & Chandler, 1993). While variations in kin relationship are well documented in the descriptive literature, most of the interventions above do not identify or address the specific needs of adult children, spouses, or other family relationships within their protocols. The effectiveness or efficacy of the programmatic approaches summarized above would likely increase if: (1) recognition of variations in kin relationship was incorporated into intervention content; and (2) protocols included more than one family member who is involved in the life of the resident following institutionalization, since involving these individuals in the overall intervention approach could prove most beneficial to boosting family involvement. Recognizing the multiple configurations of families may help to refine and facilitate staff-family care plans and relationships, and in some cases prove integral to the successful involvement of not only a primary family member, but the entire family as well.

Diversity. A common limitation in caregiving research is the lack of ethnic, racial, and socioeconomic diversity in recruited samples. The lack of diversity in samples often severely limits the generalizability of results and weakens any conclusions of effectiveness. Moreover, given the variation in family structure and caregiving processes often found in families of diverse origin (whether it be ethnically, racially, or economically; see Dilworth-Anderson, 2001), it is important to develop intervention strategies that are flexible and encompass this diversity prior to implementing programs in routine practice. For example, research on older adults among various racial and ethnic groups (such as African-Americans) has indicated that informal help exchanged within diverse families involves various types of caregiving structures (i.e., different combinations of 'primary,' 'secondary,' and 'tertiary' caregivers; see review by Dilworth-Anderson, Williams, & Gibson, 2002). Moreover, prior descriptive research has emphasized the culturally explicit rules and guidelines families of diverse race and ethnicity apply to the care provided to older adults as well as the interactions between caregivers, other family members, and various social institutions. Studies have identified the values related to reciprocity, filial obligation, and sense of responsibility that characterizes caregiving in diverse racial and ethnic contexts (e.g., sense of reliance on extended kin networks), and that cultural assessments of the illnesses or diseases of the elderly relative (e.g., viewing a loved one with dementia as having "bad blood") shape how assistance is provided to the care recipient (Dilworth-Anderson et al., 2002). Future interventions that move beyond the traditional conceptualization of the 'primary caregiver → care recipient' for diverse families and incorporate measures of family structure and cultural meaning could offer significant refinement to existing programs that have been evaluated among predominately Caucasian samples.

Attrition. As indicated above, attrition in resident, family, or staff samples is often an unavoidable challenge facing researchers who attempt to evaluate interventions for family members of chronically impaired older adults. Although attrition in long-term care samples is largely unavoidable due to the functional and cognitive impairment of residents (particularly among NH samples), any evaluations that attempt to measure longer-term outcomes of family-based interventions must likely consider the effects of extensive attrition. As recommended by Stark, Kane, Kane, and Finch (1995), several strategies can be included to counteract the effects of attrition bias in long-term care samples. For example, in addition to a model of participants who remain in the analysis, parallel models including residents who both remain in the study over time as well as those who exit can be compared. Residents who die can be assigned the lowest values on measures of importance. Although this approach may be overly stringent, it certainly can address the potentially negative effects of attrition. As recommended by Heckman and others (Berk, 1983; Heckman, 1979; Miller & Wright,

1995), several empirical approaches can also be incorporated to counteract the effects of attrition bias in longitudinal evaluations, such as the Heckman two-stage approach (Heckman, 1979). The Heckman adjustment involves modeling the 'decision' to leave a longitudinal evaluation. The statistical information about each person's likelihood of exiting the study (i.e., the Mills ratio) can then be included as an 'attrition adjuster' to correct for bias in empirical models.

Theoretical refinement. Interventions designed to improve family involvement following NH placement are largely atheoretical. Strong conceptual models are needed to identify the antecedents and ramifications of family involvement in residential long-term care and guide the development of interventions in these situations. For example, a potential model of family involvement in residential long-term care that captures elements of caregiving stress and dynamics prior to placement as well as descriptive findings on the types and ramifications of family involvement (e.g., see Davis & Buckwalter, 2001; Naleppa, 1996) may prove particularly effective in conceptually grounding subsequent research. An important component of such models should be time, as family-resident relationships have their genesis in lives prior to placement (Kelley, Swanson, Maas, & Tripp-Reimer, 1999). These experiences in addition to prospective events must be considered when analyzing and intervening on behalf of families during and long after placement.

Practice Recommendations

Multi-component approaches. Research on psychosocial interventions for family caregivers in the community consistently concludes that multifaceted programs which provide individualized services are more effective than most commonly designed caregiver interventions that emphasize only education and support (Schulz, O'Brien, Czaja, Ory, Norris, & Martire, 2002). This literature review builds on these prior findings by further emphasizing the need for multi-component approaches when enhancing family adaptation and involvement following the institutionalization of an elderly relative. As the programs by Maas et al. (2000) and Pillemer and colleagues (2003) suggest, strategies that combine support with more individually tailored components (e.g., staff meetings with individual family members to formulate care plans) represent the state-of-the-art in family-based intervention in long-term care. Further identification of components that are useful when intervening on behalf of families will continue to refine the trend towards multi-component strategies. Such research will also help to promote the need for interventions that are flexible and tailored to the diverse needs of caregiving families.

Several conceptual tools are available to practitioners that can guide the development of more complex, multi-component intervention approaches, such as family life education (FLE) principles. The main goal of FLE is to strengthen and enrich individuals and family well-being (e.g., Arcus, 1992; Brubaker & Roberto, 1992). Family-based intervention strategies within the FLE framework could emphasize the following: (1) the quality and continuity of family relationships prior to, during, and after placement; (2) understanding how individuals and families have managed stressful situations in the past when developing strategies to improve family adaptation to the institutionalization experience; (3) the implementation of approaches that involve multiple family members across generations who are likely to visit and remain integrated in the resident's life, such as grandchildren; (4) reliance on families and residents themselves as informational resources to guide individualized care plans; and (5) the recognition that variations in gender, kin relationship, and racial/ethnic background demands flexible programs in contrast to the 'one intervention fits all' approach. Multi-component family-based programs in long-term care that incorporate FLE guidelines may prove even more effective than past interventions for facilities, staff, families, and residents.

Timing. There is a paucity of approaches that alleviate the potential upheaval that may affect families during and immediately after placement of an older relative in a NH. Locating a suitable NH, notifying and preparing the care recipient for the transition, and coping with the subsequent emotional issues often place significant stress upon the entire family (Dellasega & Mastrian, 1995). Unfortunately, practical interventions and support programs are often inadequate or non-existent, leaving families to navigate the long-term care system without the support and assistance of a trained professional (Dellasega & Mastrian, 1995; Ryan & Scullion, 2000). While some existing interventions to promote family involvement following institutionalization may help address the needs of families of newly admitted residents (e.g., Peak, 2000), there is a clear gap in service availability for family members just beginning to manage the ramifications of NH placement. Evaluations of strategies designed to assist family members of newly admitted residents would provide a clearer contribution to the literature and serve as an integrative scientific bridge with family-based interventions oriented to improve family involvement and family-staff relationships.

Incorporation of multiple stakeholder perspectives. Programs that appear to exert the greatest impact consider multiple stakeholders when attempting to increase and facilitate family involvement. For example, interventions that incorporate family and staff in collaborative partnerships/contracts have reported efficacy in improving family involvement in some areas (e.g., Anderson et al., 1992; Maas et al., 2000; Pillemer et al., 2003). In addition to assessing the benefits of these programs for family/staff relationships, these interventions could measure potential outcomes for residents and the facility environment more consistently in order to document the overall ramifications of family-based intervention programs. In particular, it appears that the success of family involvement interventions depends on the culture of each facility (e.g., Caron et al., 1999). It is likely that the divergent or convergent views of social workers, families, residents, and staff may influence the overall effectiveness of a given intervention, and practitioners must take steps to ensure that programs are flexible enough to develop services and activities that address the complex interrelationships between these key individuals. To date, we know little about whether the overall goals of particular interventions mesh with those of important stakeholders. Future evaluations that document the interactive relationship between program implementation and facility environment/culture over time and how various stakeholders disagree or work together would help practitioners determine which approaches are most feasible in their respective facilities.

In particular, measurement from the resident's perspective has been notably lacking. Current statistics suggest that 50-75% of NH residents are suffering from dementia (Magaziner, German, Zimmerman, Hebel, Burton, Gruber-Baldini, May, & Kittner, 2000). It is generally assumed that researchers have a difficult, if not impossible, time administering open-ended or closed-ended measures that collect reliable information on key resident outcome measures, such as quality of life. However, an increasing number of studies are recognizing that dementia patients, even in more severe stages of the disease, can provide reliable information on their mood and quality of life (Brod, Stewart, Sands, & Walton, 1999; Lawton, van Haitsma, & Klapper, 1996; Logsdon, Gibbons, McCurry, & Teri, 1999). These methods could be adapted and included in future evaluations to more effectively discern the role of family-based interventions in improving resident outcomes.

CONCLUSION

Family caregiving of disabled older adults is in many respects a career, with the institutionalization of the relative a key transition. As interventions have emerged to promote family involvement and family-staff relationships in residential long-term care, a number of important issues remain in the literature. Future evaluations that recognize the complexity and diversity of the family care context and adopt rigorous methodological designs will refine current strategies to assist families. In addition, programs that have multiple components and consider a variety of stakeholder perspectives will help facilitate the widespread implementation of effective programs. In this manner, family-based interventions will achieve increased levels of success following the institutionalization transition.

REFERENCES

Anderson, K. H., Hobson, A., Steiner, P., & Rodel, B. (1992). Patients with dementia: Involving families to maximize nursing care. *Journal of Gerontological Nursing, 18*, 19-25.

Aneshensel, C. S., Pearlin, L. I., Mullan, J. T., Zarit, S. H., & Whitlatch, C. J. (1995). *Profiles in caregiving: The unexpected career.* San Diego: Academic Press.

Arcus, M. E. (1992). Family life education: Toward the 21st century. *Family Relations, 41*, 390-393.

Berk, R. A. (1983). An introduction to sample selection bias in sociological data. *American Sociological Review, 48*, 386-398.

Brod, M., Stewart, A. L., Sands, L., & Walton, P. (1999). Conceptualization and measurement of quality of life in dementia: The Dementia Quality of Life instrument (DQoL). *The Gerontologist, 39*, 25-35.

Brubaker, T. H. & Roberto, K. A. (1992). Family life education for the later years. *Family Relations, 42*, 212-221.

Cantor, M. H. (1983). Strain among caregivers: A study of experience in the United States. *The Gerontologist, 23*, 597-604.

Caron, W., Hepburn, K., Luptak, M., Grant, L., Ostwald, S., & Keenan, J. (1999). Expanding the discourse of care: Family constructed biographies of nursing home residents. *Families, Systems, & Health, 17*, 323-335.

Cox, C. & Ephross, P. H. (1989). Group work with families of nursing home residents: Its socialization and therapeutic functions. *Journal of Gerontological Social Work, 13*, 61-73.

Davis, L. L. & Buckwalter, K. (2001). Family caregiving after nursing home admission. *Journal of Mental Health and Aging, 7*, 361-379.

Dellasega, C. & Mastrian, K. (1995). The process and consequences of institutionalizing an elder. *Western Journal of Nursing Research, 17*(2), 123-140.

Dilworth-Anderson, P. (2001). Family issues and the care of persons with Alzheimer's disease. *Aging & Mental Health, 5*, S49-S51.

Dilworth-Anderson, P., Williams, I. C., & Gibson, B. E. (2002). Issues of race, ethnicity, and culture in caregiving research: A 20-year review. *The Gerontologist, 42*, 237-272.

Fabisewski, K. J. & Howell, M. C. (1986). A model for family meetings in the long term care of Alzheimer's disease. *Journal of Gerontological Social Work, 9*, 113-117.

Gaugler, J. E., Kane, R. L., Kane, R. A., Clay, T., & Newcomer, R. (2003). Predicting institutionalization of cognitively impaired older people: Utilizing dynamic predictors of change. *The Gerontologist, 43*, 219-229.

Gaugler, J. E., Zarit, S. H., & Pearlin, L. I. (1999). Caregiving and institutionalization: Perceptions of family conflict and socioemotional support. *International Journal of Aging and Human Development, 49*, 15-38.

Grau, L., Teresi, J., & Chandler, B. (1993). Demoralization among sons, daughters, spouses, and other relatives of nursing home residents. *Research on Aging, 15*, 324-345.

Greenfield, W. L. (1984). Disruption and reintegration: Dealing with familial response to nursing home placement. *Journal of Gerontological Social Work, 8*, 15-21.

Hansen, S. S., Patterson, M. A., & Wilson, R. W. (1988). Family involvement on a dementia unit: The Resident Enrichment and Activity Program. *The Gerontologist, 4*, 508-511.

Heckman, J. J. (1979). Sample selection bias as specification error. *Econometrica, 47*, 153-161.

Helphand, M. & Porter, C. M. (1982). The family group within the nursing home: Maintaining family ties of long-term care residents. *Journal of Gerontological Social Work, 4*, 51-62.

Hepburn, K. W., Caron, W., Luptak, M., Ostwald, S., Grant, L., & Keenan, J. M. (1997). The Families Stories Workshop: Stories for those who cannot remember. *The Gerontologist, 37*, 827-832.

Kelley, L. S., Swanson, E., Maas, M. L., & Tripp-Reimer, T. (1999). Family visitation on special care units. *Journal of Gerontological Nursing, 25*, 14-21.

Kiely, D. K., Simon, S. E., Jones, R. N., & Morris, J. N. (2000). The protective effect of social engagement on mortality in long-term care. *Journal of the American Geriatrics Society, 48*, 1367-1372.

Lawton, M. P., van Haitsma, K., & Klapper, J. (1996). Observed affect in nursing home residents with Alzheimer's disease. *Journal of Gerontology: Psychological Sciences, 51B*, P3-P14.

Linsk, N. L., Miller, B., Pflaum, R., & Ortigara-Vick, A. (1988). Families, Alzheimer's disease, and nursing homes. *Journal of Applied Gerontology, 7*, 331-349.

Logsdon, R. G., Gibbons, L. E., McCurry, S. M., & Teri, L. (1999). Quality of life in Alzheimer's disease: Patient and caregiver reports. *Journal of Mental Health and Aging, 5*, 21-32.

Maas, M. L., Swanson, E., Buckwalter, K. C., Lenth, R., Specht, J. P. et al. (2000). *Nursing interventions for Alzheimer's family role trials: Final report* (No. RO1NR01689). Iowa City: University of Iowa.

Magaziner, J., German, P., Zimmerman, S. I., Hebel, J. R., Burton, L., Gruber-Baldini, A. L., May, C., & Kittner, S. (2000). The prevalence of dementia in a statewide sample of new nursing home admissions age 65 and over: Diagnosis by expert panel. *The Gerontologist, 40*, 663-672.

Marsden, A. M. (1990). Education for support of nursing home residents. *Journal of Extension, 28*, 1-6. Available: *http://www.joe.org/joe/1990fall/a2.html*.

Miller, R. B. & Wright, D. W. (1995). Detecting and correcting attrition bias in longitudinal family research. *Journal of Marriage and the Family, 57*, 921-929.

Mittelman, M. S., Epstein, C., & Pierzchala, A. (2003). *Counseling the Alzheimer's caregiver*. United States: The American Medical Association.

Naleppa, M. J. (1996). Families and the institutionalized elderly: A review. *Journal of Gerontological Social Work, 27*, 87-111.

National Citizens' Council for Nursing Home Reform (1998). *Family education and outreach: Final report*. Retrieved 5/10/2003, from http://www.nccnhr.org/pdf/REPORT598.pdf

Numerof, R. E. (1983). Building and maintaining bridges: Meeting the psychosocial needs of nursing home residents and their families. *The Clinical Gerontologist, 1*, 53-67.

Palmer, D. S. (1991). Co-leading a family council in a long-term care facility. *Journal of Gerontological Social Work, 16*, 121-134.

Peak, T. (2000). Families and the nursing home environment: Adaptation in a group context. *Journal of Gerontological Social Work, 33*, 51-66.

Penrod, J. D., Kane, R. A., & Kane, R. L. (2000). Effects of post-hospital informal care on nursing home discharge. *Research on Aging, 22*, 66-82.

Pillemer, K., Suitor, J. J., Henderson, C. R., Meador, R., Schultz, L., Robison, J., & Hegeman, C. (2003). A cooperative communication intervention for nursing home staff and family members of residents. *The Gerontologist, 43 Special Issue II*, 96-106.

Ryan, A. A. & Scullion, H. F. (2000). Nursing home placement: An exploration of the experiences of family caregivers. *Journal of Advanced Nursing, 32*(5), 1187-1195.

Safford, F. (1980). A program for families of the mentally impaired elderly. *The Gerontologist, 20*, 656-660.

Sancier, B. (1984). A model for linking families to their institutionalized relatives. *Social Work, 29*, 63-67.

Schoenberg, N. E., Amey, C. H., Stoller, E. P., & Muldoon, S. B. (in press). Lay referral patterns involved in cardiac treatment seeking among middle-aged and older adults. *The Gerontologist*.

Schulz, R., O'Brien, A., Czaja, S., Ory, M., Norris, R., Martire, L. M. et al. (2002). Dementia caregiver intervention research:. *The Gerontologist, 42*, 589-602.

Schumacher, K. L. (1995). Family caregiver role acquisition: Role-making through situated interaction. *Scholarly Journal for Nursing Practice, 9*, 211-226.

Shulman, M. D. & Mandel, E. (1988). Communication training of relatives and friends of institutionalized elderly persons. *The Gerontologist, 28*, 797-799.

Sidell, N. L. (1997). Easing transitions: Solution focused principles and the nursing home resident's family. *Clinical Gerontologist, 18*, 21-41.

Stark, A. J., Kane, R. L., Kane, R. A., & Finch, M. (1995). Effect on physical functioning of care in adult foster homes and nursing homes. *The Gerontologist, 35*, 648-655.

Stone, R., Cafferata, G. L., & Stangl, J. (1987). Caregivers of the frail elderly: A national profile. *The Gerontologist, 27,* 616-626.

Tennstedt, S. L., McKinlay, J. B., & Sullivan, L. M. (1989). Informal care for frail elders: The role of secondary caregivers. *The Gerontologist, 29,* 677-683.

Van Meter, M. J. S. & Johnson, P. (1985). Family decision making, long-term care for the elderly and the role of religious organizations: Part III: Interventions for religious professionals and organizations. *Journal of Religion & Aging, 1,* 73-88.

Vinton, L., Mazza, N., & Kim, Y-S. (1998). Intervening in family-staff conflicts in nursing homes. *The Clinical Gerontologist, 19,* 45-68.

Whitlatch, C. J. & Noelker, L. (1996). Caregiving and caring. *Encyclopedia of Gerontology, 1,* 253-268.

Relationship Quality with Parent, Daughter Role Salience, and Self-Esteem of Daughter Caregivers

Lydia Wailing Li
Marsha Mailick Seltzer

SUMMARY. This study examined the effects of two aspects of relationship quality with parent (relationship strain and affective closeness) on daughter caregivers' self-esteem, and whether their effects are moderated by daughter role salience. Cross-sectional data from 137 married daughter caregivers with children were analyzed. Hierarchical regression analysis shows that relationship strain has negative effects on the daughters' self-esteem, regardless of daughter role salience, whereas the positive effects of affective closeness on self-esteem are stronger for

Lydia Wailing Li is Assistant Professor, School of Social Work, University of Michigan, 1080 S. University, Ann Arbor, MI 48109-1106. Marsha Mailick Seltzer is Director of Waisman Center and Professor, School of Social Work, University of Wisconsin-Madison, Madison, WI.

Address correspondence to: Lydia Wailing Li, Assistant Professor, School of Social Work, University of Michigan, 1080 S. University, Ann Arbor, MI 48109-1106 (E-mail: lydiali@umich.edu).

Preparation of this manuscript was supported by a grant from the National Institute on Aging (R01 AG09388). The authors are grateful to Berit Ingersoll-Dayton for reviewing an earlier draft of the manuscript, Stephanie Unangst, Jane Rafferty, and Terri Torkko for technical and editorial assistance, Barbara Larson and Renee Makuch for coordinating the data collection, and the Wisconsin Bureau on Aging for providing access to the sample on which this article is based.

[Haworth co-indexing entry note]: "Relationship Quality with Parent, Daughter Role Salience, and Self-Esteem of Daughter Caregivers." Li, Lydia Wailing, and Marsha Mailick Seltzer. Co-published simultaneously in *Marriage & Family Review* (The Haworth Press, Inc.) Vol. 37, No. 1/2, 2005, pp. 63-82; and: *Challenges of Aging on U.S. Families: Policy and Practice Implications* (ed: Richard K. Caputo) The Haworth Press, Inc., 2005, pp. 63-82. Single or multiple copies of this article are available for a fee from The Haworth Document Delivery Service [1-800-HAWORTH, 9:00 a.m. - 5:00 p.m. (EST). E-mail address: docdelivery@haworthpress.com].

daughters whose daughter role is salient than for those less salient. The findings have implications for how practitioners can help married daughters manage relationship strain with their parents, examine the personal meaning of their daughter role, and bolster their own self-esteem while engaged in parent care. *[Article copies available for a fee from The Haworth Document Delivery Service: 1-800-HAWORTH. E-mail address: <docdelivery@haworthpress.com> Website: <http://www.HaworthPress.com> © 2005 by The Haworth Press, Inc. All rights reserved.]*

KEYWORDS. Caregiving, intergenerational relationships, identity salience

INTRODUCTION

Past research has suggested that adult women with a surviving parent are likely to become caregivers to their parents (Brody, 1985; Himes, 1994). Numerous studies have examined the stress of parent care on adult daughters' well-being, indicated by depressive symptoms, anxiety, and physical health (e.g., Dura, Stukenberg, & Kiecolt-Glaser, 1991; Li, Seltzer, & Greenberg, 1999). Relatively few, however, have investigated specifically whether the parent care experience influences the self-esteem of adult daughters, although self-esteem has often been employed as an unmeasured construct in interpretations of the stress-distress process (Lee & Shehan, 1989; Thoits, 1991).

In this study, we investigate whether the quality of the relationship with the parent in a caregiving context is associated with the self-esteem of daughter caregivers. To assess the quality of relationship, we examine two aspects of relationship quality between daughters and parents: affective closeness and relationship strain. Further, we examine whether the salience of the daughter role moderates the association between these two aspects of relationship quality and the daughters' self-esteem.

To explore how the caregiving context may influence self-esteem, we will utilize identity theory and the life course perspective. Theorists have suggested that the self-concept is composed of multiple identities (Rosenberg, 1979; Stryker, 1980). *Identities* refer to self-in-role meanings and "are claimed and sustained in reciprocal role relationships" (Thoits, 1983, p. 175; Atkinson, 1989). Stryker (1980) notes that identities within the self-concept are organized hierarchically on the basis of salience. The more salient identities are those that the individual values more, and which would, if threatened, have more detrimental effects on the self-concept. The idea of identity salience is similar to the concept of psychological centrality proposed by Rosenberg (1979). Indeed, Rosenberg and Pearlin (1978) illuminate how self-esteem is related to central vs. peripheral axes of self-concept in the following passage:

> Some elements of the self-concept are at the center of attention, at the heart of the individual's major concerns, others are at the periphery. . . . Thus, the impact of any given component on global self-esteem will depend on its importance or unimportance, centrality or periphery, in the individual's cognitive structure. (p. 67)

In relation to our parents, each of us has a child identity. According to the life course perspective, the salience of the child identity within an individual should vary across the life span (Atkinson, 1989). For instance, among young girls, the child (daughter) identity may be a primary component of their self-concept because few other identities have developed. As women enter adulthood and acquire other social roles, such as wife and mother, the psychological importance of the daughter identity may decrease. However, when the parent becomes dependent and needs care, the salience of the daughter identity may again emerge, partly because of increased interactions with the parent during caregiving, and partly because of the threat of losing the parent (Cicirelli, 1991). In other words, in a caregiving context, the daughter's self-esteem may be more sensitive to the relationship with her parent, due to the increased salience of the daughter identity, which the caregiving context brings to the fore.

Indeed, past studies of the general population have shown a concurrent association between the psychological well-being of adult children and relationship quality with their aging parents (Barnett, Kibria, Baruch, & Pleck, 1991; Umberson, 1992; Welsh & Stewart, 1995), suggesting that parents continue to play a significant role in adult children's lives. Studies of adult child caregivers have also shown that a better relationship with the parent care recipients is related to more caregiving effectiveness, and less caregiving stress, burden, and depressive symptoms of adult child caregivers (Carpenter, 2001; Townsend & Franks, 1995; Walker, Martin, & Jones, 1992).

IDENTITY SALIENCE HYPOTHESIS

Although the daughter identity may be more salient at the stage when the parent needs care compared to other periods of adulthood, individual variations among daughter caregivers in the salience of the daughter role are expected, as accumulating literature suggests that individuals differ in the importance they attach to the roles they occupy (Krause, 1994; Thoits, 1992). As mentioned earlier, theorists have argued that experiences encountered in relation to a salient role would have a stronger psychological impact than those related to a less salient role. This proposition has been referred to as *identity salience hypothesis* and has been tested in a number of past studies, mostly in the context of role stress (Krause, 1994; Martire, Stephens, & Townsend, 2000; Simon, 1992; Thoits, 1992). Mixed support for this hypothesis has been reported, however. For instance, Simon found that salience of the parental identity increases one's vulnerability to parental strains, but Thoits (1992) did not find identity salience to moderate the effect of perceived stress in a role-identity domain on psychological distress.

While spanning different roles, these past studies have one distinct thread in common: they have focused on stressful or negative role experiences in testing the identity salience hypothesis. Whether and how the effects of positive role experience are conditioned by identity salience, however, have rarely been examined. If identity salience increases one's vulnerability to role stress because it threatens a valued aspect of self (Burke, 1991; Thoits, 1991), then it should amplify one's benefit from positive role experience because a valued aspect of one's self-concept is affirmed. To our knowledge, this amplification hypothesis has not been tested in previous studies.

RELATIONSHIP QUALITY WITH PARENT

In the present study, we examine both the positive and negative aspects of the daughter-parent relationship, as experienced by daughter caregivers. The positive aspect refers to the daughter's feelings of closeness to her parent, and the negative aspect refers to the daughter's feelings of strain in the interaction with the parent. A close parent-child relationship has been suggested as indicating a strong attachment bond, and should provide the daughter a sense of security and comfort, as well as affirmation of self (Atkinson, 1989). A close relationship with the parent is also socially valued and reinforced.

On the contrary, relationship strain with the parent is against social norms regarding parent-child relationships. To daughter caregivers, in particular, the increased interactions associated with a strained parent relationship may serve as an uncomfortable reminder of the tension resonating within the daughter identity. Here, we address the extent to which daughter caregivers' feelings of closeness and strain in the relationship with their parents are associated with their self-esteem, and the moderating role of daughter role salience in the association between these two aspects of relationship quality and self-esteem.

HYPOTHESES

Four hypotheses are tested in this study.

1. Relationship strain is negatively associated with the self-esteem of daughter caregivers.
2. The negative association of relationship strain and self-esteem is stronger for daughters whose daughter role is highly salient than those less salient.
3. Affective closeness is positively associated with the self-esteem of daughter caregivers.
4. The positive association of affective closeness and self-esteem is stronger for daughters whose daughter role is highly salient than those less salient.

METHODS

Sample

The data for this analysis were taken from the second wave of a longitudinal study of women in Wisconsin entitled Well-Being of Women (WBW). We focused on the Wave 2 point of data collection because the question about daughter role salience was not asked at Wave 1.

The WBW study sample was recruited through a probability sampling procedure. In 1991, using random-digit dialing procedures, the State of Wisconsin Bureau on Aging identified two probability samples: 2,250 persons aged 60 or older, and 500 persons younger than 60 who provided care to a relative older than 60. To ensure a sufficiently large pool of caregivers for the study, the base was supplemented with an additional 1,000 households, also obtained through random-digit dialing procedures. For additional details about the sampling plan, see Li, Seltzer, and Greenberg (1999).

We telephoned these persons in 1993 to determine their current caregiving status. A daughter was classified as a caregiver if she provided assistance to a parent, aged 60 or older, due to his or her aging or disability, with at least one of the following tasks: housework, preparing meals, managing finances, yard work, shopping, taking medications, getting around inside the house, eating, dressing, bathing, using the toilet, getting in and out of bed, and remembering things. Of those who met the study criteria, 79.3% agreed to participate.

At Wave 1, 211 daughters with living biological parents were interviewed. By Wave 2, 37 parents had died and 5 daughters refused to be re-interviewed, leaving 169 daughters in the WBW study. For the present analysis, we selected only daughters who were also mothers and were married at Wave 2. We made this decision for two reasons: First, the vast majority of the WBW sample were married (85%) and had children (92%); and second, the measure of daughter role salience was based on a question that asked about perceptions of important family roles. To limit the study sample to daughter caregivers who were married and were mothers ensured that all sample members occupied the same primary family roles, thereby reducing the possibility of measurement artifact. Consequently, the final sample for this analysis was 137.

Table 1 presents the characteristics of the study sample. The daughters averaged 59 years of age. Virtually all were white (96%). Fewer than half (45%) had attended college and about half (50%) were employed. Their average household income in 1995 was $47,737. The daughters had provided care to their parents for an average of 8 years and about 4% were caring for both parents.

The parents of these daughters averaged 85 years old, and were mostly mothers (84%). The majority were widowed (80%) and only 17% were still married. The parents had various major conditions that resulted in the need for care, such as Alzheimer's disease (22%), arthritis (11%), heart trouble (10%), walking difficulty (7%), and blindness (6%). Most of the parents (56%) lived in their own homes, about one-fifth (21%) lived in a nursing home or institutional setting, and only a minority (6%) lived with their daughter caregivers.

TABLE 1. Sample Characteristics

Characteristics of Daughters	
Age (mean years)	58.8
White (%)	95.6
Education (%)	
< high school	6.6
high school graduate	54.7
some college	29.2
bachelor's degree or more	16.1
Employed (%)	50.4
Income (mean $)	47,737
Duration of care (mean years)	8.2
Caring for both parents (%)	3.6
Characteristics of Parents	
Age (mean years)	85.2
Female (%)	84.0
Marital status (%)	
Married	16.8
Widowed	80.3
Divorced	2.9
Reason for care (%)	
Alzheimer's disease	21.8
Arthritis	11.3
Heart trouble	9.8
Walking difficulty	6.8
Blindness	6.0
Others	44.3
Living arrangement (%)	
Own home	56.2
Nursing home	21.2
With daughter caregiver	5.8
Others	16.8

Data Collection and Measures

Data were collected by personal interviews with the daughters, primarily in their homes. The key study variables were measured as follows:

Relationship Strain. Five items from the Zarit Burden Interview (Zarit, Reever, & Bach-Peterson, 1980) were used to indicate strains in the relationship between the daughter caregiver and her parent. These five items asked the daughter the extent to which she felt strained, angry, guilty, resentful, and nervous or depressed in the interaction with her parent. Each item was rated from not at all (1) to extremely (3). The relationship strain measure was obtained through an exploratory factor analysis using Wave 1 data and a confirmatory factor analysis using Wave 2 data (data available from the first author). The alpha reliability of the relationship strain scale in this sample was .86.

Affective Closeness. Affective closeness with the parent was assessed with 5 items from the Positive Affect Index, which has been used widely in studies of intergenerational relationships (Bengtson & Black, 1973). The items ask how much the daughter understands, trusts, is fair to, respects, and has affection for her parent. Each item was rated from not at all (1) to extremely (6). Alpha reliability of the affective closeness scale in this sample was .83.

Daughter Role Salience. Daughter caregivers were asked to list and rank up to 3 of their most important family roles at the time. Almost half of the daughters (46%) did not include the role of daughter in any of these roles. This skewed distribution led us to dichotomize the daughter role salience variable, with coding 1 for daughters who included the daughter role in their important family roles and 0 for those who did not.

Control Variables. Our decision about control variables was informed by previous literature (Harter, 1990; Lee & Shehan, 1989; Reitzes & Mutran, 1994) as well as preliminary data analysis. Correlation coefficients were computed between self-esteem and 20 background variables, including socio-demographic variables of the daughters (e.g., age, education, income, employment status, grandmother status), their level of social participation and marital satisfaction, as well as the parents' socio- demographic characteristics (e.g., gender, living arrangement) and impairment levels (e.g., cognitive limitations, behavioral problems). Background variables that had a significant correlation ($p < .05$) with self-esteem were included as control variables. Consequently, four variables were chosen: Education, measured dichotomously (0 = no college, 1 = some college or more); grandmother status (0 = no grandchildren, 1 = one or more grandchildren); self-rated health from 1 = poor to 4 = excellent; and marital satisfaction which was measured with an index of 17 items from the Marital Satisfaction Questionnaire for Older Persons (Haynes, Floyd, Lemsky, Rogers, Winemiller, Heilman, Werle, Murphy, & Cardone, 1992). Each item was rated from very dissatisfied (1) to very satisfied (6). The scale had an alpha of .97.

Self-Esteem. The dependent variable, self-esteem, was measured by the Rosenberg Self-Esteem Scale (Rosenberg, 1965). The scale consists of 10 items that require respondents to report feelings about the self. A sample item is "I feel I have a number of good qualities." Each item was rated on a 4-point Likert scale from strongly disagree (1) to strongly agree (4). The alpha reliability of the scale was .87.

Data Analysis

Zero-order correlation was used to examine the bivariate relationships of all study variables, with particular interest in the correlation between the two dimensions of relationship quality with parent (i.e., relationship strain and affective closeness). We also compared the two groups of daughters–those for whom the daughter role was salient and those for whom it was not salient–on all study variables. To examine the main and moderating effects of the two dimensions of relationship quality and daughter role salience, hierarchical linear regression was conducted. Relationship strain and affective closeness were analyzed in separate models first, due to their high correlation. Three successive blocks of independent variables were entered to predict the self-esteem of daughter caregivers: first control variables and daughter role salience (Model 1), then relationship quality variable, as measured by either relationship strain or affective closeness (Model 2), and lastly, a multiplicative term of relationship quality $\times$ daughter role salience (i.e., either relationship strain $\times$ daughter role salience or affective closeness $\times$ daughter role salience) (Model 3). The two relationship quality variables were centered before forming the multiplicative terms (Aiken & West, 1991). The main effects of relationship quality on the daughter's self-esteem were tested in Models 2, while the moderating effects of daughter role salience were tested in Models 3. In order to examine whether the two dimensions of relationship quality have independent effects on self-esteem, we also conducted an analysis with both relationship strain and affective closeness as simultaneous predictors of self-esteem, which was reported after the separate analyses. Note that our use of the term *effects* in this study implies associations rather than causal relationships, as our data are cross-sectional in nature.

RESULTS

Descriptive Findings

Table 2 presents the mean and standard deviation of each study variable, as well as the zero-order correlation among them. Note that the

TABLE 2. Means, Standard Deviations, and Zero-Order Correlations of Study Variables (N = 137)

	1	2	3	4	5	6	7	M (SD)
1. Self-esteem	–							34.48 (4.63)
2. Relationship strain	−.28**	–						6.85 (2.01)
3. Affective closeness	.17	−.66**	–					24.90 (3.68)
4. Daughter role salience	−.03	.03	−.15	–				.46 (.50)
5. Education	.22**	−.11	.03	−.02	–			.45 (.50)
6. Grandma	.21*	.01	−.03	.12	−.11	–		.62 (.49)
7. Health	.17*	−.10	−.03	.15	.03	.07	–	3.06 (.63)
8. Marital satisfaction	.24**	−.10	.18*	−.04	−.00	.04	.18*	81.02 (16.60)

Note. *p < .05; **p < .01 (2-tailed)

means of relationship strain (6.85 out of a possible range of 5-15) and affective closeness (24.90 out of a possible range of 5-30) are at the low and high end of their scales, respectively, which suggests that most daughters feel more positively than negatively in the relationship with their parents. When using the means of relationship strain and affective closeness to divide our sample into high and low levels in each of these variables, we found a mixed pattern of feelings toward their parents among the daughters: 45% were high in closeness and low in strain, 29% high in strain and low in closeness, 15% high in closeness and high in strain, and 11% low in closeness and low in strain.

The two dimensions of relationship quality–relationship strain and affective closeness with parent–have a relatively high negative correlation (r = −.66), suggesting that they are dependent on each other. Yet each has some unique variance that is not shared by the other. Both dimensions of relationship quality are correlated with self-esteem of the daughters. Daughter role salience, however, is not correlated significantly with self-esteem, nor with either dimension of relationship quality. We compared the two groups of daughters (i.e., daughter role salient and daughter role not salient) on all study variables and the 20 background variables used to determine control variables mentioned earlier (e.g., daughter's age and employment status, parent's cognitive limitations and behavioral problems) and found that they do not differ significantly on any of these variables (results not shown here).

Relationship Strain with Parent and Self-Esteem of Daughter Caregivers

We conducted multiple regression analysis to examine the main effects of relationship strain on the daughters' self-esteem, and whether its effects are moderated by daughter role salience, controlling for education, grandmother status, self-rated health, and marital satisfaction of the daughters. The results are presented in Table 3. Model 1 has only the control variables and daughter role salience as predictors. In Model 2 the relationship strain variable was added, which is statistically significant and explains an additional 5% of the variance of the daughters'

TABLE 3. Effects of Relationship Strain with Parent on Self-Esteem of Daughter Caregivers

Independent Variables	Model 1		Model 2		Model 3	
	b (s.e.)[a]	β[b]	b (s.e.)	β	b (s.e.)	β
Education (1 = some college or more)	2.23 (.74)**	.24	2.01 (.73)**	.21	1.94 (.73)**	.21
Grandma (1 = grandmother)	2.16 (.77)**	.23	2.16 (.75)**	.23	2.16 (.75)**	.23
Health (1-4, poor to excellent)	.87 (.61)	.12	.73 (.59)	.10	.81 (.60)	.11
Marital satisfaction	.06 (.02)*	.21	.05 (.02)*	.19	.05 (.02)*	.19
Daughter role salience (1 = salient)	.59 (.75)	.06	.51 (.73)	.06	.53 (.73)	.06
Relationship strain	–	–	–.52 (.18)**	–.23	–.35 (.24)	–.25
Relationship strain X Daughter role salience	–	–	–	–	–.40 (.37)	–.09
R^2	.17		.22		.23	
ΔR^2			.05**		.01	

Note. *p < .05; **p < .01 (2-tailed)
[a]Unstandardized regression coefficients (standard errors)
[b]Standardized regression coefficients. The Friedrich (1982) approach was used to obtain the standardized solutions, as suggested by Aiken and West (1991) for regression equations that involve interaction terms.

self-esteem. The multiplicative term, relationship strain × daughter role salience, was added in Model 3 and is not statistically significant. F-ratio test indicates that Model 3 is not significantly different from Model 2. Thus, the results do not support the identity salience hypothesis; rather, relationship strain has negative effects on the daughters' self-esteem, regardless of the salience of the daughter role. Other predictors of self-esteem include education, grandmother status, and marital satisfaction of the daughter–daughters who have college or more education, are grandmothers, and are more satisfied with their marital relationship have higher self-esteem.

Affective Closeness with Parent and Self-Esteem of Daughter Caregivers

The multivariate analysis of affective closeness is presented in Table 4. Following the same procedure used for relationship strain, we first examined the main effect of affective closeness on self-esteem (Model 2)

TABLE 4. Effects of Affective Closeness with Parent on Self-Esteem of Daughter Caregivers

Independent Variables	Model 1		Model 2		Model 3	
	b (s.e.)[a]	β[b]	b (s.e.)	β	b (s.e.)	β
Education (1 = some college or more)	2.23 (.74)**	.24	2.20 (.74)**	.24	2.17 (.72)**	.23
Grandma (1 = grandmother)	2.16 (.77)**	.23	2.17 (.76)**	.23	2.22 (.75)**	.23
Health (1-4, poor to excellent)	.87 (.61)	.12	.91 (.60)	.12	1.06 (.59)	.14
Marital satisfaction	.06 (.02)*	.21	.05 (.02)*	.19	.05 (.02)*	.18
Daughter role salience (1 = salient)	.59 (.75)	.06	.43 (.75)	.05	.44 (.74)	.05
Affective closeness	–	–	.16 (.10)	.13	−.05 (.13)	.18
Affective closeness X Daughter role salience	–	–	–	–	.51 (.20)*	.20
R²	.17		.19		.23	
ΔR²			.02		.04*	

Note. *p < .05; **p < .01 (2-tailed)
[a]Unstandardized regression coefficients (standard errors)
[b]Standardized regression coefficients. The Friedrich (1982) approach was used to obtain the standardized solutions, as suggested by Aiken and West (1991) for regression equations that involve interaction terms.

and found that to be statistically non-significant. The multiplicative term of affective closeness and daughter role salience, which was entered into Model 3, is statistically significant. An F-test indicates that Model 3 explains more of the variation (an additional 4%) in daughters' self-esteem than Model 2. The results therefore suggest that the effects of affective closeness on the daughters' self-esteem vary, depending on the salience of the daughter role.

We used the procedure suggested by Aiken and West (1991) to plot the interaction effect of affective closeness and daughter role salience. Figure 1 depicts the slope of self-esteem on affective closeness for the two groups of daughters (daughter role salient vs. daughter role not salient). We used the self-esteem scores at low (one standard deviation below the mean), mean, and high (one standard deviation above the mean) levels of affective closeness, to construct the regression lines for the two groups. As shown, for daughters with salient daughter role, a closer relationship with their parents is associated with higher self-esteem (standardized regression coefficient, $\beta = .36^{**}$), whereas for those whose daughter role is not salient, affective closeness has minimal effects on their self-esteem. ($\beta = -.04$, *ns*).

Simultaneous Effects of Relationship Strain and Affective Closeness on Self-Esteem

When both relationship strain and affective closeness were entered into the model to predict the daughters' self-esteem, a similar pattern of

FIGURE 1. Moderating Effects of Daughter Role Salience in the Association of Affective Closeness with Parent and Self-Esteem of Daughter

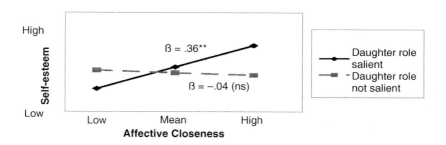

Note: **p < .01; ns = not significant at p < .05.
β = Standardized regression coefficients.

results as reported above was observed. Table 5 presents the simultaneous analysis.

Model 1 shows that the main effect of relationship strain is statistically significant, whereas that of affective closeness is not, which is consistent with the results when each dimension of relationship quality was analyzed separately. However, the standard errors of the coefficients of relationship strain and affective looseness are much larger, compared to the main effect models with only one dimension of relationship quality in the model, which suggests that multicollinearity may be an issue.

The interaction effect of relationship strain and daughter role salience was tested in Model 2 and is not statistically significant, whereas the interaction effect of affective closeness and daughter role salience,

TABLE 5. Simultaneous Effects of Relationship Strain and Affective Closeness on Self-Esteem

Independent Variables	Model 1		Model 2		Model 3	
	b (s.e.)[a]	β[b]	b (s.e.)	β	b (s.e.)	β
Education (1 = some college or more)	1.99 (.73)**	.21	1.93 (.73)**	.21	1.94 (.71)**	.21
Grandma (1 = grandmother)	2.16 (.75)**	.23	2.15 (.75)**	.23	2.21 (.73)**	.23
Health (1-4, poor to excellent)	.69 (.60)	.09	.79 (.61)	.11	.83 (.59)	.11
Marital satisfaction	.06 (.02)*	.20	.05 (.02)*	.19	.05 (.02)*	.19
Daughter role salience (1 = salient)	.56 (.74)	.06	.56 (.74)	.06	.59 (.72)	.06
Relationship strain	−.58 (.24)*	−.25	−.40 (.30)	−.27	−.65 (.24)**	−.28
Affective closeness	−.05 (.14)	−.04	−.04 (.14)	−.03	−.31 (.16)	−.01
Relationship strain X Daughter role salience	−	−	−.39 (.37)	−.08	−	−
Affective closeness X Daughter role salience	−	−	−		.56 (.20)*	.22
R^2	.22		.23		.27	
ΔR^2			.01[c]		.05*[c]	

Note. *p < .05; **p < .01 (2-tailed)
[a]Unstandardized regression coefficients (standard errors)
[b]Standardized regression coefficients. The Friedrich (1982) approach was used to obtain the standardized solutions, as suggested by Aiken and West (1991) for regression equations that involve interaction terms.
[c]Change of R^2 as compared to Model 1.

tested in Model 3, is significant. Both findings are consistent with those reported before. Overall, this simultaneous analysis suggests that relationship strain with the parent has negative effects on the self-esteem of daughters, independent of daughter role salience and affective closeness (as well as education, grandmother status, health, and marital satisfaction). In contrast, affective closeness has stronger positive effects on the self-esteem of daughters who value the role of daughter highly as opposed to those who do not, net of the effects of relationship strain and other control variables.

DISCUSSION

Our findings suggest that the self-esteem of daughter caregivers is associated with both relationship strain and affective closeness with the parent. On one hand, the negative effects of relationship strain are uniform across all daughters, regardless of the salience of the daughter role. On the other hand, the positive effects of affective closeness are conditioned by daughter role salience, with greater benefits for daughters whose daughter role is salient than for those for whom the role is less salient. Thus, the findings partially support the identity salience hypothesis that daughter role salience amplifies the positive effects of affective closeness with the parent, but do not support the hypothesis in relation to relationship strain. These findings are consistent with a previous study that did not find parent care centrality to moderate the effect of parent care stress (Martire et al., 2000). However, this study has advanced the literature by examining the moderating role of identity salience in relation to positive role experience. Our findings suggest that identity salience increases the psychological benefits that one can derive from positive role experience, possibly because a valued aspect of the self is validated and affirmed (Welsh & Stewart, 1995).

Studies of social relationships have suggested that the detrimental effects of negative social exchanges are greater than the beneficial effects of positive social exchanges (Rook, 1990). To some extent, our findings support this assertion, as the negative effects of relationship strain on self-esteem are uniform, whereas the positive effects of affective closeness are conditioned by daughter role salience. However, the stronger impact of negative exchanges than positive exchanges may be truer for some groups than others. Our analysis shows that for daughters whose daughter role is salient, the effects of relationship strain on self-esteem ($\beta = -.23^{**}$) are not greater than that of affective closeness ($\beta = .36^{**}$), whereas for daughters whose daughter role is not salient, the stronger detrimental impact of relationship strain ($\beta = -.23**$ vs. $\beta = -.04$, ns, for affective closeness) is obvious. Future research on the impact of positive and negative social exchanges may need to consider the subjective importance that individuals attach to different role relationships.

Implications for Practice

Our findings have implications for professionals working with older families. With the increase of life expectancy, more women will assume the role of parent care. While much attention has been given to caregiver burden and distress, our study suggests that caregiving needn't be viewed solely as a negative predicament. Rather, our study suggests the view that parent care offers an opportunity for daughters to improve their sense of self, as well as one that poses risk for devaluation of the self. From this perspective, practitioners working with caregiving families may focus on strengthening the salient components of the self-concept of daughter caregivers. Indeed, past studies have shown that self-esteem is an important psychological resource that buffers the negative effects of stress on physical and mental health (Seeman, Berkman, Gulanski, Robbins, Greenspan, Charpentier, & Rowe, 1995; Shamir, 1986). Thus, helping daughter caregivers to preserve and increase positive self-evaluation should be a priority.

Our findings suggest that relationship strain is a major correlate of the daughters' negative self-assessment, therefore, reducing strains in the daughter-parent relationship should be a goal of intervention. An early study showed that a cognitive-behavioral intervention that assisted adult daughters with widowed mothers to reduce unrealistic expectations of their responsibility for their mothers and to interact with them in a manner that promotes the mother's self-reliance was effective in decreasing the daughters' feelings of burden and increasing their positive feelings towards their mothers (Scharlach, 1987). This may be a promising approach when working with daughter caregivers, especially those who experience high levels of relationship strain with their parents. The negative effects of relationship strain on the self-esteem of daughter caregivers appear to be ubiquitous, at least not conditioned by the salience of the daughter role, suggesting the need to develop more effective strategies to manage such strains in the caregiving context.

At the same time, helping professionals should build on the strength of the daughter-parent relationship and help adult daughters to maximize the benefits they can derive from the parent care experience. Our findings suggest that those who feel close to their parent and attach great importance to the role of daughter are more likely to have a positive self-assessment. Thus, helping daughter caregivers to examine the personal meaning of the daughter role, as well as appreciate their feelings of closeness to their parents, may be effective strategies to bolster their self-esteem.

Our descriptive findings suggest that the majority of daughter caregivers experienced the relationship with their parents quite positively with few strains, which challenges the stereotype of daughter caregivers and suggests the need for careful individualized assessment when working with caregiving families. In particular, practitioners should recognize the variety of feelings that daughters may have toward their parents. For instance, our data suggests that some daughters may be ambivalent (high in both closeness and strain) and some may feel detached (low in both closeness and strain) in relating to their parents. Separate assessment of the positive and negative dimensions of the daughter-parent relationship would help to detect more complex feelings.

In sum, our study suggests that parent care can be an opportunity for growth for adult daughters, although it also poses risks. Careful assessment of the daughter's experience, especially feelings of strain and closeness with their parents, as well as the salience of the daughter role would help professionals to develop individualized care plans that promote positive self-concept and reduce the risk of negative self-assessment for daughter caregivers.

Strengths and Limitations

This study employed a sample of daughter caregivers who were themselves mothers and were married to examine the effects of both positive and negative interactions with parent on the self-esteem of daughters, and the extent to which the effects of each dimension of relationship quality are conditioned by daughter role salience. The study sample was based on a larger sample of daughter caregivers recruited through a probability sampling procedure, which has an advantage over previous studies that relied on samples recruited through advertisements or organizations. However, the study has several methodological caveats that should be noted.

First, our sample was predominately white, which is characteristic of the older population in Wisconsin. The generalization of our findings to other racial/ethnical group therefore is not warranted. Second, this sample of married daughter caregivers with children does not represent daughter caregivers who are unmarried and/or not parents. Although we found the same pattern of results in an additional analysis with all daughter caregivers in the larger study, the predominance of married daughters with children in this larger sample prevents us from generalizing the findings to other daughters. Third, our sample size is relatively small which may have limited the statistical power to test our hypotheses. Overall, the study speaks to the importance of assessing the quality of the relationship between daughter caregivers and their parent care recipients, especially in terms of its relevance to the self-esteem of daughters. Our study suggests that in order to help daughter caregivers to maximize the benefits and minimize the negative effects of parent care, the positive and negative dimensions of the daughter-parent relationship should be differentiated, and the salience of the daughter role should be examined.

REFERENCES

Aiken, L. & West, S. (1991). *Multiple regression: Testing and interpreting interactions.* Thousand Oaks, CA: Sage.

Atkinson, M. P. (1989). Conceptualizations of the parent-child relationship: Solidarity, attachment, crescive bonds, and identity salience. In J. A. Manicini (Ed.), *Aging parents and adult children* (pp. 81-98). Lexington, MA: Lexington Books.

Barnett, R. C., Kibria, N., Baruch, G. K., & Pleck, J. H. (1991). Adult daughter-parent relationships and their association with daughters' subjective well-being and psychological distress. *Journal of Marriage and the Family, 53,* 29-42.

Bengtson, V. L. & Black, K. D. (1973). Inter-generational relations and continuities in socialization. In P. Baltes & K. W. Schaie (Eds.), *Life-span development psychology: Personality and socialization* (pp. 207-234). New York: Academic Press.

Brody, E. M. (1985). Parent care as a normative family stress. *Gerontologist, 25(1),* 19-29.

Burke, P. (1991). Identity process and social stress. *American Sociological Review, 56,* 836-849.

Carpenter, B. (2001). Attachment bonds between adult daughters and their older mothers: Associations with contemporary caregiving. *Journal of Gerontology: Psychological Sciences, 56B,* 257-267.

Cicirelli, V. (1991). Attachment in old age: Protection of the attached figure. In K. Pillemer & K. McCartney (Eds.), *Parent-child relations throughout life* (pp. 25-42). Hillsdale, NJ: Erlbaum.

Dura, J., Stukenberg, K., & Kiecolt-Glaser, J. (1991). Anxiety and depressive disorders in adult children caring for demented parents. *Psychology and Aging, 6,* 467-473.

Friedrich, R. J. (1982). In defense of multiplicative terms in multiple regression equations. *American Journal of Political Science, 26,* 797-833.

Harter, S. (1990). Causes, correlates, and the functional role of global self-worth: A life-span perspective. In R. J. Sternberg & J. Kolligian, Jr. (Eds.), *Competence considered* (pp. 67-97). New Haven, CT: Yale University Press.

Haynes, S. N., Floyd, F., Lemsky, C., Rogers, E., Winemiller, D., Heilman, N., Werle, M., Murphy, T., & Cardone, L. (1992). The marital satisfaction questionnaire for older persons. *Psychological Assessment, 4,* 473-482.

Himes, C. (1994). Parental caregiving by adult women: A demographic perspective. *Research on Aging, 16,* 191-211.

Krause, N. (1994). Stressors in salient social roles and well-being in later life. *Journal of Gerontology, 49,* 137-148.

Lee, G. & Shehan, C. (1989). Social relations and the self-esteem of older persons. *Research on Aging, 11,* 427-442.

Li, L. W., Seltzer, M. M., & Greenberg, J. S. (1999). Change in depressive symptoms among daughter caregivers: An 18-month longitudinal study. *Psychology and Aging, 14,* 206-219.

Martire, L. M., Stephens, M. A. P., & Townsend, A. L. (2000). Centrality of women's multiple roles: Beneficial and detrimental consequences for psychological well-being. *Psychology and Aging, 15,* 148-156.

Reitzes, D. C. & Mutran, E. J. (1994). Multiple roles and identities: Factors influencing self-esteem among middle-aged working men and women. *Social Psychology Quarterly, 57,* 313-325.

Rook, K. (1990). Stressful aspects of older adults' social relationships: Current theory and research. In Stephens, M., Crowther, J., Hobfoll, S., & Tennenbaum, D. (Eds.), *Stress and coping in later-life families* (pp. 173-192). New York: Hemisphere.

Rosenberg, M. (1965). *Society and the adolescent self-image.* Princeton, NJ: Princeton University Press.

Rosenberg, M. (1979). *Conceiving the self.* New York: Basic Books.

Rosenberg, M. & Pearlin, L. (1978). Social class and self-esteem among children and adults. *American Journal of Sociology, 84,* 53-78.

Scharlach, A. (1987). Relieving feelings of strain among women with elderly mothers. *Psychology and Aging, 2,* 9-13.

Seeman, T., Berkman, L., Gulanski, B., Robbins, R., Greenspan, S., Charpentier, P., & Rowe, J. (1995). Self-esteem and neuroendocrine response to challenge: MacArthur studies of successful aging. *Journal of Psychosomatic Research, 39,* 69-84.

Shamir, B. (1986). Self-esteem and the psychological impact of unemployment. *Social Psychology Quarterly, 49,* 61-72.

Simon, R. (1992). Parental role strains, salience of parental identity, and gender differences in psychological distress. *Journal of Health and Social Behavior, 33,* 25-35.

Stryker, S. (1980). *Symbolic interactionism.* Menlo Park: Benjamin/Cummings.

Thoits, P. (1983). Multiple identities and psychological well-being: A reformulation and test of the social isolation hypothesis. *American Sociological Review, 48,* 174-187.

Thoits, P. (1991). On merging identity theory and stress research. *Social Psychology Quarterly, 54,* 101-112.

Thoits, P. A. (1992). Identity structures and psychological well-being: Gender and marital status comparisons. *Social Psychology Quarterly, 55,* 236-256.

Townsend, A. & Franks, M. (1995). Binding ties: Closeness and conflict in adult children's caregiving relationships. *Psychology and Aging, 10,* 343-351.

Umberson, D. (1992). Relationships between adult children and their parents: Psychological consequences for both generations. *Journal of Marriage and the Family, 54,* 664-674.

Walker, A., Martin, S., & Jones, L. (1992). The benefits and costs of caregiving and care receiving for daughters and mothers. *Journal of Gerontology: Social Sciences, 47*, S130-139.

Welsh, W. M. & Stewart, A. J. (1995). Relationships between women and their parents: Implications for midlife well-being. *Psychology and Aging, 10*, 181-190.

Zarit, S. H., Reever, K. E., & Bach-Peterson, J. (1980). Relatives of the impaired elderly: Correlates of feelings of burden. *Gerontologist, 20*, 649-655.

Paying Family Caregivers:
An Effective Policy Option
in the Arkansas Cash and Counseling
Demonstration and Evaluation

Lori Simon-Rusinowitz
Kevin J. Mahoney
Dawn M. Loughlin
Michele DeBarthe Sadler

Lori Simon-Rusinowitz is Research Director, Cash and Counseling Demonstration and Evaluation, University of Maryland Center on Aging, 2360 HHP Bldg., College Park, MD 20742. Kevin J. Mahoney is National Project Director, Cash and Counseling Demonstration and Evaluation, Boston College Graduate School of Social Work, McGuinn Hall, Room 306, 140 Commonwealth Avenue, Chestnut Hill, MA 02467-3807 (E-mail: kevin.mahoney@bc.edu). Dawn M. Loughlin is Senior Researcher, University of Maryland Center on Aging 2360 HHP Bldg., College Park, MD 20742 (E-mail: d.shoop@verizon.net). Michele DeBarthe Sadler, MPH, is Faculty Research Assistant, University of Maryland Center on Aging, 1240E HHP Bldg., College Park, MD 20742 (E-mail: cheleds@comcast.net).

Address correspondence to: Lori Simon-Rusinowitz, Research Director, Cash and Counseling Demonstration and Evaluation, University of Maryland Center on Aging, 2360 HHP Bldg., College Park, MD 20742 (E-mail: Ls119@umail.umd.edu).

The CCDE is co-sponsored by the Robert Wood Johnson Foundation (RWJF) and the U.S. Department of Health and Human Services, Office of the Assistant Secretary for Planning and Evaluation (DHHS/ASPE). The Centers for Medicare and Medicaid Services (CMS) granted 1115 research and demonstration waivers to the Demonstration states, and provides continuing oversight and technical assistance.

[Haworth co-indexing entry note]: "Paying Family Caregivers: An Effective Policy Option in the Arkansas Cash and Counseling Demonstration and Evaluation." Simon-Rusinowitz, Lori et al. Co-published simultaneously in *Marriage & Family Review* (The Haworth Press, Inc.) Vol. 37, No. 1/2, 2005, pp. 83-105; and: *Challenges of Aging on U.S. Families: Policy and Practice Implications* (ed: Richard K. Caputo) The Haworth Press, Inc., 2005, pp. 83-105. Single or multiple copies of this article are available for a fee from The Haworth Document Delivery Service [1-800-HAWORTH, 9:00 a.m. - 5:00 p.m. (EST). E-mail address: docdelivery@haworthpress.com].

SUMMARY. Informal family assistance is often a key factor in determining whether a person with a disability can live in a community setting. However, the practice of paying relatives as caregivers remains controversial. This article reports findings from the Cash and Counseling Demonstration and Evaluation (CCDE) in Arkansas, in which consumers receive a cash allowance to purchase personal assistance services. In this comparison of consumers who hired family vs. non-family workers, consumers who hired relatives received more service and had equal or superior satisfaction and health outcomes, as compared to those who hired non-relatives. Findings are further clarified by drawing from worker focus group reports and program experience, and policy issues are specifically addressed. *[Article copies available for a fee from The Haworth Document Delivery Service: 1-800-HAWORTH. E-mail address: <docdelivery@haworthpress.com> Website: <http://www.HaworthPress.com>* © 2005 by The Haworth Press, Inc. All rights reserved.]*

KEYWORDS. Paying family caregivers, consumer direction

INTRODUCTION

The critical role of families in providing care to elders and younger persons with disabilities is well established. Nearly one in four U.S. households are involved in this type of informal (unpaid) care (National Alliance for Caregiving, 1997). Family members comprise more than 70% of caregivers of older persons with activity limitations, and the vast majority (76%) of caregivers are unpaid (Super, 2002). Informal caregivers, usually female family members, provide assistance with activities of daily living, including eating, bathing, dressing, using the toilet, and transferring from bed to chair. Informal caregivers also provide assistance with varied household tasks such as laundry and meal preparation. These types of assistance are often key factors in determining whether a person with disabilities can live in a community setting (Stone, 1995). In addition, the national economic value of informal caregiving labor is great–estimated in 1997 to be $196 billion (Arno, Levine, & Memmott, 1999).

Findings from the 1997 National Caregiver Survey indicate that family caregivers who provide these critical services tend to have multiple responsibilities. About two-thirds of family caregivers in this country are working and 41% have one or more children under 18 years old living in their household. The average family caregiver provides care 18 hours per week, while about 1 in 5 provide care at least 40 hours per week (National Alliance for Caregiving, 1997). Despite the important role, economic value and multiple responsibilities of family caregivers, the practice of paying relatives who provide this critical care is considered controversial in this country. Opponents of paying family caregivers raise the issues of appropriate public-private responsibility, quality of care, fraud and abuse, and fears of exploding public costs for services primarily provided for free (Blaser, 1998; Linsk, Keigher, Simon-Rusinowitz, & England, 1992). Proponents of paying family caregivers speak to benefits of the approach, such as increasing consumer choice, improving the quality of care, and expanding the limited worker supply (Linsk et al., 1992; Simon-Rusinowitz, Mahoney, & Benjamin, 1998).

This debate about the advantages and disadvantages of paying family caregivers has also become more important with research showing the effects of caring for a disabled relative on family employment and on retirement income. Findings from a 1995 survey conducted by The Arc show that 52% of families indicated that someone in their family had turned down or quit a job to provide care for their disabled family member (cited in Agosta & Melda, 1995). In addition to losing income, these family caregivers also lose out on earning important Social Security benefits. Because Social Security benefits are determined by an individual's employment income, unpaid caregivers may receive severely limited benefits. Without Social Security, family caregivers are more vulnerable to becoming impoverished as they themselves age (Kijakazi, 2002). As the majority of family caregivers are female, women bear the brunt of the negative consequences of unpaid family caregiving.

While the policy debate about the advantages and disadvantages of paying family caregivers has continued for many years, it has become especially relevant in the context of the growing concern about the limited direct care labor force. A recent nationwide survey found that recruiting and retaining direct care workers was a major workforce issue for 42 states (Yamada, 2002). Projections of increased demand for services needed by aging baby boomers, combined with decreasing numbers of traditional workers (i.e., women aged 25-54) indicate the need for expansion of the direct care workforce (Wilner, 2000). Increased interest in consumer-directed services that allow consumers to hire their own workers are likely to increase demand for workers. In addition, implementation of the Olmstead decision (Olmstead: 527 U.S. 581, 1999), which encourages states to provide community-based long-term services for persons with a disability, are likely to do the same.

RESEARCH ON PAID FAMILY CAREGIVING

In 1985, Linsk and colleagues studied payments to family caregivers in the Illinois Community Care Program as an effort to guide Illinois policy makers and leaders in determining whether this caregiving arrangement should be expanded, modified, or discontinued (Linsk et al., 1992). This research found varying levels of policy support, with the majority of the respondents speaking of the advantages of the policy for consumers and their families, including better quality care, improved consumer satisfaction and economic benefits for consumers and families. Other research on payments to family caregivers has also primarily addressed policy and program issues, including the extent of such payment programs and their features (Gerald, 1993; Linsk, Osterbusch, Keigher, & Simon-Rusinowitz, 1986; England, Linsk, Simon-Rusinowitz, & Keigher, 1989; Burwell, 1986), attitudes of administrators and policy makers about family payments (Linsk et al., 1986), consumer-directed homecare approaches, including family providers (Sabatino, 1990), family payments as an incentive to caregivers (Biegel, 1986), and evaluation of specific programs (Whitfield & Krompholz, 1981).

While much research addresses policy and program issues, there is also a body of research that discusses the views of consumers and family care providers. A 1997 evaluation of the California In-Home Supportive Services program reported that about half of the consumers in the consumer-directed model hired relatives and a quarter hired friends. Those consumers who hired relatives tended to be older, less educated and more likely to come from ethnic and racial minorities than other consumer-directed model clients. They also on average felt less risk and felt more secure than those cared for by others. They indicated having more choice about how their services were delivered as well as having more satisfaction about the choice they had, in comparison to clients who did not hire family members. Consumers hiring relatives and friends rated them as more reliable than workers who were strangers. They also felt interpersonally closer to their workers than clients who hired non-family providers (Benjamin, Matthias, & Franke, 1998). Similarly, a 1996 study of elderly Medicaid personal care recipients in Michigan, Texas, and Maryland found that client satisfaction was related to consumers having the choice of who provides their personal care, and to having the ability to hire family, friends, and neighbors as their caregivers (Doty, Kasper, & Litvak, 1996).

Background research for the Cash and Counseling Demonstration and Evaluation, which permits hiring relatives as workers, has offered similar support for paying family caregivers (Mahoney, Simon-Rusinowitz, Loughlin, Desmond, & Squillace, 2002). Between 90% and 92% of the respondents to a four state telephone survey indicated that they would be interested in a consumer-directed cash option because of the ability to "hire whomever you wanted to provide services, even a friend or relative." Participants in follow-up focus groups in four states agreed that the option of hiring relatives or friends as their personal care worker was a positive program feature, although reactions were mixed about doing so. A few of the focus group participants were concerned with the possibility of a lower level of professionalism from family members and an ability to deal comfortably with provider-client conflicts. However, most focus group participants liked the idea of being able to pay a friend or family member who was already helping with personal care needs. In addition, consumers felt that their relatives would know their special needs, likes, and dislikes better. Focus group participants also shared that being able to hire a relative or friend would allow consumers to hire someone of the same ethnicity. This last finding appears to be an especially important factor for African-American and Hispanic consumers.

As research shows, paying family caregivers and the more general idea of consumer-directed services are two concepts that tend to be linked. Consumers interested in consumer-directed services have expressed a preference for the ability to hire family and friends as workers, and when these consumers are able to direct their own services they do, in practice, tend to hire family and friends. Similarly, consumers who hire their own workers, including family and friends, conduct employer responsibilities, such as hiring, firing, and supervising workers. The present study also links these issues in its comparison of paid family and non-family caregivers in a consumer-directed setting.

THE PRESENT STUDY

The Cash and Counseling Demonstration and Evaluation (CCDE) is a test of one of the most unfettered forms of consumer-directed services–offering Medicaid consumers in Arkansas, Florida, and New Jersey a cash allowance and information services in lieu of agency-delivered care. CCDE clients can use their cash benefit to purchase personal care services, assistive devices, or home modifications that best meet their individual needs. Information services include assistance with cash management tasks such as hiring, training, and managing workers as well as payment responsibilities. In theory, consumers who shop for the most cost-effective providers may then (through such savings) have funds to purchase additional services (Kapp, 1996).

The CCDE, which will be completed in 2005, compares cost, quality, and satisfaction of consumers receiving traditional personal care services with those receiving the cash option. The evaluation is co-sponsored by the Robert Wood Johnson Foundation (RWJF) and the U.S. Department of Health and Human Services, Office of the Assistant Secretary for Planning and Evaluation (DHHS/ASPE). It operates under section 1115 Research and Demonstration waivers granted by the Centers for Medicare and Medicaid Services (CMS). Primary quantitative data collection and analysis is being conducted by Mathematica Policy' Research, Inc. For a detailed description of the CCDE design, please refer to Mahoney, Simone, and Simon-Rusinowitz (2000).

This current analysis is based on CCDE data from Arkansas, the first state in which CCDE data has been collected. This analysis is a comparison of related and non-related clients and workers within the consumer-directed cash option group. Specifically, we are comparing the: (1) background characteristics of both consumers who hired a relative vs. a non-relative, and workers who worked for relatives vs. non-relatives, (2) types and amounts of service provided and received by related and non-related clients and workers, and (3) health and satisfaction outcomes for related and non-related clients and workers. The discussion will be augmented with findings from focus groups conducted with paid workers in Arkansas, as well as general CCDE Arkansas experience.

METHODS

Volunteer enrollment for the CCDE Arkansas study, the Arkansas IndependentChoices Program, began in December 1998 and ended in April 2001. At enrollment, clients who felt that they may be unable or unwilling to individually handle the tasks associated with the consumer-directed Independent Choices program, were asked to appoint a program representative–usually a family member or friend, to assist with these responsibilities if necessary.

Clients were randomly assigned to consumer-directed (n = 1004) and traditional service (n = 1004) groups. Traditional service clients were given a list of home health care agencies that they could contact for their personal assistance services, or, if they were currently receiving services, they could continue to rely on their previous agencies. The clients in the consumer-directed group were given a monthly allowance and were responsible for procuring their personal assistance services on their own. Consumer-directed clients could hire whomever they wanted for their personal assistance, with the exception of spouses, or the person acting as their program representative. The amount of the monthly allowance was determined by the number of personal assistance hours in the client's existing care plan, or, for new clients, the number of hours in the care plan as determined by enrollment nurses. The monthly benefit for consumer-directed clients in Arkansas averaged $320 per month.

Consumer-directed clients had the option to use fiscal intermediaries to handle bookkeeping and payroll services on their behalf, and almost all clients chose to use these free services. Counselors were also available, at no charge to the consumer, to provide advice and support for creating cash management plans and for recruiting and hiring workers. Counselors also approved cash management plans, and monitored the program for fraud and abuse. Consumer-directed clients were free to dis-enroll from the study at any time and return to traditional services. Clients were surveyed at enrollment (prior to randomization), at four months and at nine months, with computer-assisted telephone interviews. Experienced MPR interviewers were trained on the specific surveys. Clients who were unable or unwilling to answer for themselves could provide proxy respondents to answer the surveys for them. In these cases, interviewers asked that the "most knowledgeable person" complete the telephone survey. During the 9-month survey, respondents were asked to provide names and contact information for their primary paid workers. For a detailed description of data collection methods and procedures see Foster, Brown, Phillips, Schore, and Carlson (2003).

Samples

The current analysis compares outcomes for clients who chose to hire a family worker versus clients who chose to hire a non-family worker, as well as outcomes for those two types of workers–when clients had a choice of workers to hire. We therefore limited our focus to the consumer-directed clients, and their paid family or paid non-family workers.

Client Sample. Attempts were made to survey clients or their proxy respondents at all survey points, even if the client had dis-enrolled (n = 189) from the program or was deceased (n = 32), and 885 clients or proxy respondents from the consumer-directed group (88%) completed the 9-month survey. Of the 885 respondents, 636 respondents were participating in the program and paying a worker at the time of the nine-month survey. For clients with multiple paid workers we could not determine if responses applied to a family or non-family worker, due to the structure of the survey. We therefore further restricted this analysis to clients with only one worker. We included 436 clients in this analysis; 334 clients who were paying one family worker (182 of these had proxy respondents), and 102 clients who were paying one non-family worker (49 of these had proxy respondents). Clients over age 65 were more likely to be dis-enrolled from the study and, if participating, more likely to have had multiple paid workers. Thus, the clients in our analysis sample, which was drawn from 9-month Independent Choices participants with one worker, were slightly younger than the original volunteer sample (64% age 65 or older vs. 72% age 65 or older).

Questions about client satisfaction and quality of care were only asked of clients who responded for themselves, and of proxy respondents who were not also paid workers. For these questions, this analysis sample consists of 215 clients (or their non-worker proxy respondents) who were currently paying one family worker and 88 clients (or their non-worker proxy respondents) who were currently paying one non-family worker.

Worker Sample. Based on client referrals from the 9-month survey, 248 primary paid workers who were not primary informal caregivers at baseline were contacted, and 216 of these workers completed the paid worker survey. During a separate survey of primary informal caregivers who were identified at baseline, an additional 125 respondents were identified as paid (although not necessarily primary paid) workers. Another 175 workers who were identified as primary informal caregivers at baseline were identified again during the 9-month client survey as primary paid workers. Both of these groups also completed survey items that applied to paid workers. We included all three of these groups of consumer-directed paid workers in this analysis, which resulted in a sample of 417 paid family workers and 99 paid non-family workers.

Although the client and the worker analysis samples are drawn from the same treatment group pool, they are not necessarily dyads or matched sets of clients and workers. In some cases a client's worker could not be contacted, and in eleven cases two paid workers were working for the same client (only one identified as primary). Since even workers for the same client may have had very different responses, levels of satisfaction, backgrounds or outcomes, in general, all paid worker respondents are included in the paid worker analyses. Questions concerning worker satisfaction and assistance with tasks were restricted to those who were identified as the primary (though not necessarily only) paid worker. For these questions, the sample consists of 306 family workers identified as the primary paid worker and 85 non-family workers identified as the primary paid worker.

RESULTS

Sixty-four percent of the clients in our analysis sample were over 65 years of age, and 77% were female. Clients could choose more than one racial category, and thus the racial percentages total more than 100%. Specifically, 60% identified as white, 37% identified as Black, and 5% identified as American Indian or Alaskan Native. Less than 1% each identified as Asian or other. Clients received an average of 25.2 hours of paid care over a two-week period.

The majority of paid workers in our analysis sample were female (88%), but younger than the client sample; the majority of workers were between 35 and 54 years of age. The racial percentages were similar to the client sample–63% identified as white, 35% identified as Black and 5% identified as American Indian/Alaskan Native. Fifty-three percent of the paid workers were married, 37% had children under 18 years of age, and 68% had graduated from high school.

Client Characteristics

Table 1 presents characteristics of clients who hired a family worker versus clients who hired a non-family worker. Clients who hired a family worker were more likely to be living with others and to have had previous unpaid help in the week prior to baseline. These clients were less likely to have had previous paid help, and also less likely to have had both paid and unpaid help, in the week prior to baseline. American Indian/Alaskan Native clients made up a smaller percentage than would be expected of those who hired a family member. That is, 11% of clients who hired non-family identified as American Indian/Alaskan Native compared to only 4% of those who hired family.

TABLE 1. Client Characteristics by Worker-Client Relationship

Client Characteristic		Clients Who Hired Family (n = 334) Column %	Clients Who Hired Non-Family (n =102) Column %
Female		79	72
Over 65		65	61
Married		17	14
Race	White vs. all other	58	66
	Black vs. all other	39	29
	American Indian or Alaskan Native vs. all other	4	11*
Living with others		69	53**
Living in rural area		37	35
Using a program rep		41	30
Self report health	Excellent	5	5
	Good	16	17
	Fair	33	29
	Poor	47	49
Help getting out of bed	Got help	30	33
	No help	68	66
	Did not get out of bed at all	2	1
Help bathing	Got help	75	72
	No help	24	28
	Did not bathe at all	1	0
Help using toilet	Got help	24	25
	No help	69	69
	Did not use at all	6	6
Unpaid help week prior to baseline		94	83**
Paid help week prior to baseline		51	71***
Both paid and unpaid help week prior to baseline		48	60*

* p < .05 *** p < .01 *** p < .001
Note: Client characteristics from non-missing responses to CCDE Arkansas baseline survey for clients participating at 9 months with only one paid worker.

Paid Worker Characteristics

Paid family workers were more likely to be female, to be married, to have known and helped the client in the past, and to be living with the client (Table 2). Workers who provided routine health care or personal care were asked if they had received training–either in a classroom,

TABLE 2. Worker Characteristics by Client-Worker Relationship

Worker Characteristic		Family Worker (n = 417) Column %	Non-Family Worker (n = 99) Column %
Female		89	80*
Worker age	15-24	9	5
	25-34	14	14
	35-44	26	23
	45-54	28	27
	55-64	16	20
	65-74	7	7
	75-84	< 1	3
Married		55	23*
Race	White	61	64
	Black	35	30
	American Indian or Alaskan Native	4	6
Helped client with routine care before hire		97	51***
Knew client before helping		100	78***
Lives with client		48	20***
Has children under 18		38	31
High school graduate		68	70
Received training in routine health care (if provided routine health care)		53	61
Received training in personal care (if provided personal care)		47	65**

* p < .05 ** p < .01 *** p < .01
Note: Worker characteristics based on non-missing responses to CCDE Arkansas paid worker survey.

from a health care professional, or formal training from the client or client's family. Family workers were less likely to report having received training in personal care.

Services Provided and Received

The surveys included two sets of measures of the service provided by workers. Clients were asked about services received from their family or non-family worker with a focus on personal care services (Table 3).

TABLE 3. Assistance Received by Client During Two-Week Reference Period by Family vs. Non-Family Paid Worker

Type of Assistance:	Percent of Clients Receiving Assistance	
	Family Paid Worker (n = 334)	Non-Family Paid Worker (n = 102)
Help with light housework/laundry	98	88***
Help doing other things	93	71***
Help around house/community	93	73***
Help with shopping	92	71***
Help with bathing or showering	90	77**
Help with other personal care	88	75**
Help taking medications	77	51***
Help with eating	67	57
Help with transportation	67	47***
Help w/routine health care	63	52**
Help getting in or out of bed	62	54
Help getting to or using toilet	60	51

** p < .01   *** p < .001
Note: Based on non-missing client responses from CCDE Arkansas 9 month client survey for participating clients with only one paid worker.

Workers were asked a different set of questions about services provided, with these questions reflecting a greater emphasis on routine health care services (Table 4). Clients with a paid family worker reported receiving equal or greater assistance on all measures of assistance. Worker reports show a similar tendency for family workers to provide equal or greater services to clients.

Clients and workers were asked similar sets of questions about the timing of care provided. Both surveys revealed that family workers were more likely to provide care during non-traditional hours such as evenings and weekends (Table 5).

Client Health and Satisfaction Outcomes

The surveys provided several measures of health and satisfaction outcomes for both consumer-directed clients and their workers. At the nine-month survey point, about 15% of clients with a family worker or a

TABLE 4. Assistance Provided by Paid Worker During Two-Week Reference Period by Family vs. Non-Family Paid Worker

	Percent Providing Assistance	
	Family Paid Worker (n = 417)	Non-Family Paid Worker (n = 99)
Type of Assistance:		
Helped with any routine health care	97	90
Helped with taking medicine	77	51***
Range of motion/other exercise	53	53
Special care of feet	42	33
Helped by checking vital signs	32	21*
Caring for pressure sores	28	19
Care of ventilator/care lung	11	9
Helped by checking blood sugar	10	6
Care of urinary catheter	6	7
Use/care of feeding tube	4	4
Care of colostomy	3	3
Helped with other routine health care	29	18*

* p < .05   ** p < .01   *** p < .001
Note: Based on non-missing worker responses from CCDE Arkansas paid worker survey.

non-family worker, when asked about their overall health, reported good or excellent versus fair or poor. There were no differences in measures of activities of daily living: difficulty taking a full bath without help, difficulty getting out of bed without help, or difficulty using the toilet or commode without help. Clients with a family or a non-family worker were also about equally likely to report taking medicine regularly (95%), and equally likely to report having a chronic health condition (89%). Ninety-seven percent of clients with a family worker and clients with a non-family worker felt that their worker had sufficient knowledge to care for their condition.

Similarly, clients with a non-family or family worker were about equally likely to report having, in the past month: shortness of breath developing or worsening (34%), forgotten medicine at least once (23%), been in a hospital or nursing home (17%), developed contractures (17%), had a urinary tract infection (15%), been injured by a paid helper (1%), or

TABLE 5. Timing of Routine Care by Family vs. Non-Family Paid Worker (as reported by clients and workers), and Mean Hours of Help Reported by Clients

	Client Survey		Worker Survey	
	Family Worker (n = 334)	Non-Family Worker (n = 102)	Family Worker (n = 417)	Non-Family Worker (n = 99)
Percent Received/Provided Help:				
Before 8:00 a.m. weekdays	56	31*	54	34*
Between 8:00 a.m.-6:00 p.m. weekdays	Not Asked	Not Asked	94	86*
After 6:00 p.m. weekdays	73	42*	76	44*
Weekends any time	88	44*	90	59*
Mean hours of help received over 2 weeks (from all sources)	Total Hours	Total Hours		
All unpaid help received	99	91		
Paid help received from worker	26	24		
All paid and unpaid help	125	115		

p < .05 chi-square analysis care provided by family vs. non-family within each survey.
Note: Based on non-missing client responses from CCDE Arkansas 9 month survey for participating clients with only one paid worker, and non-missing worker responses from CCDE Arkansas paid worker survey.

seen a doctor for a cut, burn, scald or other injury (< 1%). Clients with a family worker were, however, less likely to report a respiratory infection (26% vs. 37%, p < .05), bed sores or pressure sores (4% vs. 12%, p < .01), and having fallen (16% vs. 29%, p < .01).

Over 96% of consumer-directed clients in both groups reported that they were satisfied with how they got along with their paid worker, the time of day they got help, and the routine care, personal care and help around the house provided by their paid worker (when applicable). Clients were equally likely to report unmet need for help around the house, help with medication, and help with transportation. Clients with a family worker were more likely to be satisfied with overall arrangements for care (99% vs. 91%, p < .01), and less likely to report unmet need for personal care (22% vs. 36%, p < .05).

Worker Satisfaction

We found that paid family and non-family workers were about equally likely to report the following problems: pay delayed (35%), need for client to show more respect for the work done by the worker (16%), received less pay than earned (6%), close supervision interfered with work (5%), asked to do tasks not agreed to (2%), and disagreement concerning schedule (1%). Family and non-family primary paid workers were also about equally likely to report that they were satisfied with the feedback they were given on their performance (95%), that they liked the supervision they received (89%), and that they had a say about when to do things (91%). However, among primary paid workers, family workers were more likely to report having to hurry to complete tasks (24% vs. 11%, n = 388, p < .01). Among all paid workers for consumer-directed clients, family workers were more likely to agree that the client's family members "need to be more respectful of the work I do" (40% vs. 21%, n = 502, p < .01). Overall, however, 96% of all paid workers for consumer-directed clients felt prepared to do what was expected of them, and over 99% indicated that they were satisfied with their working conditions.

DISCUSSION AND POLICY ISSUES

The practice of paying family members who care for their relatives continues to be a controversial policy issue in this country. The findings from Arkansas clearly address policy concerns including quality of care, amount and types of services provided, as well as consumer health and satisfaction outcomes. This section will draw upon the findings reported in this article to address policymakers' frequently asked questions. Quotations from focus groups conducted with paid workers in Arkansas will be used to clarify and exemplify the results of the quantitative study. Typical policymaker issues include: reasons consumers choose to hire relatives, who will choose to hire relatives, the impact of this consumer-directed approach on consumers, informal caregivers and paid family caregivers, as well as the quality of care provided by a relative, and concerns about fraud and abuse.

Why Do Consumers Choose to Hire a Relative?

An interesting question to consider is why consumers who are given a choice frequently select relatives to provide their care? We found that a majority of our sample hired a relative as their paid worker. Research has shown that many consumers choose to hire a relative because they believe they receive better care from a person who knows and cares about them rather than a stranger. They also feel more comfortable having a trusted family member enter their home and provide intimate care than allowing a stranger to do so (Mahoney et al., 2002; Benjamin et al., 1998). Our findings support these beliefs, including reports that consumers with a paid family worker had no adverse health outcomes and fared better in some important areas, despite the fact that those relatives had less training in personal care. Consumers with paid family caregivers were also more likely to receive care during non-traditional hours, and they reported less unmet need for personal care. In a recent focus group with IndependentChoices paid workers, that primarily included paid relatives, one individual captured this point saying, "A lot of people on IndependentChoices right now are getting better care from their family members than they could ever get in any other situation" (Zacharias, 2002).

We found that Black consumers were a little more likely to hire a relative, as compared to consumers of other racial/ethnic backgrounds. This finding, although not statistically significant, is consistent with previous research (Benjamin et al., 1998). However, American Indian/Alaskan Native consumers were comparatively less likely to hire a relative. This is a clear reminder that cultures may differ in their norms and expectations, especially in such sensitive areas as family relations, health practices, and disability issues. Future research should be directed toward a more thorough investigation of these issues for minority clients.

We also found that consumers who hired family were more likely than those who hired non-family to have had previous unpaid care, and were more likely to be living with others. On the other hand, consumers who hired non-family were more likely to report previous paid care, and more likely to report both types of care. We can view these results as both a reflection of the family "connectedness" with the consumer, and as simple continuity. That is, consumers who hire family are likely to be those who have relatives ready and available to work for them; they are able to hire those relatives and many may prefer to continue a pre-existing care relationship. Consumers who hire non-family are more likely to have had a paid non-family worker available, and many may have preferred to continue that relationship. Although the data does not address this issue, it is also possible that some consumers were not able to hire their preferred worker, relative or non-relative, as that person was not available. For example, the paid worker shortage may limit the workers available to those who prefer a non-relative. However, some consumers who would prefer a relative may not have an appropriate relative to hire.

Paid Family Workers Good for Caregivers

Is a consumer-directed option that allows payments to family workers good for caregivers? For family members who struggle to balance demanding caregiving and work responsibilities, the cash option might help balance these conflicts by allowing them to work fewer hours or leave their jobs. While the average Arkansas cash benefit has been about $320 per month, this relatively small amount might provide an informal caregiver enough income to either decrease their work hours or leave an outside job. The benefit also offers the possibility of paying for respite care, another avenue to help informal caregivers juggle demanding responsibilities. A few paid family workers who took part in recent focus groups reported that they were able to quit other full-time jobs to become an IndependentChoices paid worker, but others said they were not able to decrease their regular work hours even after they became an IndependentChoices paid worker.

An added benefit for paid family workers is the opportunity to contribute to the Social Security program. Their status as a paid worker allows them to earn credits toward both disability and retirement benefits. In addition, they may be able to save some wages for retirement, an important opportunity for this primarily low-wage, female workforce. Finally, their wages provide recognition that their labor is important to their relative and to the larger community.

Policymakers worry about a "substitution effect" from this policy option, resulting in families who previously cared for a relative without pay (informally) now doing the same caregiving for pay. However, it is important to note that our findings indicate that consumers who hired a relative still received the same amount of unpaid care as those who hired non-family. In addition, in focus groups, most paid relatives reported that they had provided care prior to IndependentChoices, and that they were providing care for more hours than those for which they were paid. This would seem to negate the concern that when family members become paid workers, they will only provide care when paid. To the contrary, this finding raises a concern about family caregivers becoming overburdened by working too many hours. Twenty-four percent of the paid family workers in our sample reported having "to hurry to get things done" (vs. 11% of non-family workers). Thirty-eight percent of the paid family workers in this sample had children under 18 years of age. Future research will need to explore this "addition" effect, as much as any substitution effect. It is also important to note the many positive client outcomes associated with paying family caregivers, including increased consumer satisfaction and decreased unmet need. These outcomes may also balance policymakers' substitution effect concerns.

The current analyses show high levels of worker satisfaction among all cash option workers, family and non-family alike. Paid workers from both groups were highly satisfied with the supervision and feedback they received. Paid family workers in our sample were no more likely than non-family workers to indicate any lack of respect for their work from their clients. Clients expressed equal satisfaction with how they got along with family and non-family workers. However, paid family workers were more likely to indicate a perceived lack of respect for their work from clients' families (and presumably their own). Interestingly, IndependentChoices paid family worker focus group participants did not confirm a lack of respect from family members. Further research should explore this issue of family respect to determine what meaning it has to the family worker and to develop appropriate program supports.

In light of a concern that some family members might feel coerced into being a paid worker, especially with a labor shortage, the recent focus groups explored paid family workers' views about their positions. Of the 18 participants in the IndependentChoices paid worker focus groups, all but one had been a caregiver for the IndependentChoices client prior to the client's enrollment in the program; some for a few months or several years, others for the client's entire life. For all of them, there was no question that they would become the paid worker when the client enrolled in IndependentChoices. For some, this choice was influenced by the belief that it would be difficult finding a personal care worker willing to work for relatively low wages. For others, there were no other family members available or willing to be a caregiver. But all of these participants wanted to be the personal caregiver, and they did not report feeling obligated to accept this role. Many caregivers reported feeling "blessed" to provide care to a loved one, as indicated by the following statements from caregivers: "I think that God has put me in this position to take care of my mother at this time; my mother helped me with my children, we would've starved years ago if I didn't have my mother and it's my turn." "None of us sitting here could be doing this if God hadn't put it on our heart, . . . we're just living out what we've been called to do." "I just feel good that I'm able to be there for her right now." When asked about the challenges of being a paid caregiver, these participants acknowledged the time demands of this difficult role and the ways in which it limited their family and social lives. However, overall they appeared to accept these challenges and were happy to care for their loved ones.

Do Consumers Get Good Quality Care from a Relative?

Policymakers often express concern about the quality of care provided by family members who do not receive the same training required for agency workers. Although none of the workers in this analysis were agency workers, the non-family workers were significantly more likely to have received training in personal care. However, family worker focus group participants explained that they learned various tasks and procedures from observing home health and hospital nurses, although some noted that additional training would be helpful.

Despite differences in training, the current analysis indicates positive health and satisfaction outcomes for consumers with paid family workers, as compared with consumers with non-family workers. They reported fewer respiratory infections, bed sores or pressure sores, and falls. There were no statistically significant differences in other health or disability outcomes between clients who hired family vs. non-family. Clients with paid family caregivers reported less unmet need for personal care.

Clients were highly satisfied with both family and non-family paid caregivers; however, those with family caregivers were more satisfied with their overall care arrangements. Clients' increased satisfaction may be related to findings that paid family caregivers were more likely to work non-traditional hours, twice as likely to provide care on weekends, and they were significantly more likely to assist with numerous tasks. A statement drawn from recent focus groups with paid family caregivers indicates their experience and confidence in caring for their relatives: "we've had these family members all these years and we know what has to be done on a daily and hourly basis." Our analysis supports this view as 97% of clients (with both family and non-family workers) thought their worker had the necessary knowledge to care for them.

Cash Option Consumers

Will cash option consumers, especially those with paid family caregivers, take the cash and use it inappropriately? Will they make bad choices? Will they suffer abuse and neglect? Policymakers often worry that cash option consumers will use their cash benefit for purposes other than personal care and forego needed services. They are especially concerned about a consumer from a dysfunctional family who, for example, hires a relative with substance abuse problems and the worker squanders the cash benefit on drugs or alcohol. Our comparisons of client health and satisfaction outcomes, as well as CCDE experience to date, offer no support for this concern. While it is possible that a dysfunctional family could participate in the cash option, the CCDE States have incorporated a system of "checks and balances" (i.e., consumer representatives, bookkeeping services, as well as monitoring by counselors and fiscal intermediaries) to prevent and monitor such abuses. Contrary to policymakers' concerns about consumers with a paid family caregiver going without needed care, we find that paid family caregivers tend to provide care beyond the hours for which they are paid.

Do Paid Family Caregivers Increase the Labor Supply?

Policymakers are concerned about finding approaches to address the long-term care worker shortage. Would a policy that allows payment to family caregivers expand the limited labor supply?

Findings from this analysis, as well as CCDE experience thus far, indicate that the ability to hire family members expands the limited labor supply. At the nine-month follow-up survey, half of new recipients in the CCDE control group (i.e., those assigned to receive agency services) lacked any paid care, while the majority of cash option clients had hired at least one relative (Dale, Brown, Phillips, Schore, & Carlson, 2003). Thus, it is clear that the ability to draw upon a non-traditional labor source seems to expand the labor supply. Another important issue is that paid family caregivers have provided more flexible times during which consumers receive care. Rather than serving consumers only during traditional work hours, paid family caregivers were more likely to provide care during early morning, evening, and weekend hours.

Policymakers also want to know if this non-traditional labor source will expand the labor supply on a long-term basis (i.e., will family members only enter the labor pool to care for their relatives, or will they care for others as well). While the current analysis does not address this question, the recent focus groups explored this issue. When asked if they would consider being a personal care worker for someone other than a family member, focus group participants gave mixed reactions. Many stated that while they were comfortable providing services to a family member, they were less certain about caring for a stranger. Others might consider this possibility.

Study Limitations

Due to the survey design, this analysis was limited to clients who had only one paid worker. Clients with multiple workers may have had some differences in outcomes. Their workers may have had more respite and fewer care burdens, which could have a positive effect on the care received. However, clients with multiple workers may also experience greater inconsistencies in care. Further research should be directed toward outcomes for clients with multiple family and non-family workers.

The Arkansas IndependentChoices program does not allow clients to hire spouses as paid workers. In addition, the benefit amount in Arkansas is relatively small. These program features may impact some program outcomes, including the amounts of unpaid care that would continue when a relative is hired. In CCDE programs in New Jersey and Florida, clients may hire spouses and the benefit amounts are larger. We will learn more about these issues, as results for these states become available.

In addition, the effects of the existing shortage of personal care workers are difficult to assess. Some clients who hired a family member may have preferred to hire non-family if a worker was available. It is likely that some clients who were excluded from this comparison analysis because they had no worker at the nine-month survey point would have acquired a worker if they could. However, the shortage of personal care workers is a real life factor for clients, and this analysis sought to compare the outcomes for clients hiring family or non-family, within those real circumstances.

CONCLUSION

Overall, the experience of clients and their family workers in the consumer-directed CCDE in Arkansas appears to be quite positive in every area that has been of concern to policymakers. The majority of consumer-directed clients hired family workers, and those clients received equal or greater services, and experienced less unmet need, as compared to clients who hired non-family workers. Although two issues for family caregivers were identified, caregiver burden and respect from family members, these paid family workers reported overall high levels of satisfaction with the care arrangement. Clients who hired a family member also report superior health and satisfaction outcomes. To date in the CCDE experience, cases of fraud or abuse have been rare. We hope that these findings will inform the long-standing debate about payment to family caregivers and make this option more widely available for those who choose it.

REFERENCES

Agosta, J. & Melda, K. (1995). *Supplemental security income for children with disabilities: An exploration of child and family needs and the relative merits of the cash benefit program.* Cambridge, MA: Human Services Research Institute.

Arno, P.S., Levine, C., & Memmott, M.M. (1999). The economic value of informal caregiving. *Health Affairs, 18, 182-188.*

Benjamin, A.E., Matthias, R.E., & Franke, T. (1998). *Comparing client-directed and agency models for providing disability-related supportive services at home.* University of California, Los Angeles, School of Public Policy and Social Research.

Biegel, E. (1986). *Family elder care incentive policies: Final report of the Pennsylvania Department of Aging.* Pittsburgh: University of Pittsburgh, Center for Social and Urban Research.

Blaser, C.J. (1998). The case against paid family caregivers: Ethical and practical issues. *Generations, 22,* 65-69.

Burwell, B. (1986). *Shared obligations: Public policy influences on family care for the elderly.* (No. 55-83-0056). Cambridge, MA, SysteMetrics.

Dale, S., Brown, R., Phillips, B., Schore, J. & Carlson, B.L. (2003). The effects of Cash and Counseling on personal care services and Medicaid costs in Arkansas. *Health Affairs* Web Exclusive, November 19, 2003.

Doty, P., Kasper, J., & Litvak, S. (1996). Consumer-directed models of personal care: Lessons from Medicaid. *Milbank Memorial Fund, 74,* 37-409.

England, S.E., Linsk, N.L., Simon-Rusinowitz, L., & Keigher, S.M. (1989). Paid family caregiving and the market view of home care: Agency perspectives. *Journal of Health and Social Policy, 1,* 31-53.

Foster, L., Brown, R., Phillips, B., Schore, J., & Carlson, B. (2003). Improving the quality of Medicaid personal assistance through consumer direction: Findings from the Arkansas Cash and Counseling Demonstration. *Health Affairs,* (March 26, 2003, web exclusive).

Gerald, L. (1993). Paid family caregiving: A review of progress and policies. *Journal of Aging & Social Policy, 5,* 73-89.

Kapp, M.B. (1996). Enhancing autonomy and choice in selecting and directing long-term care services. *Elder Law Journal, 4,* 55-97.

Kijakazi, K. (2002). Impact of unreported social security earnings on people of color and women. *Public Policy and Aging Report, 12,* 9-12.

Linsk, N.L., Osterbusch, S.E., Keigher, S.M., and Simon-Rusinowitz, L. (1986). *Paid family caregiving: A policy option for community long-term care.* Final Report Submitted to Illinois Association of Family Service Agencies. Chicago, IL. University of Illinois at Chicago.

Linsk, N.L., Keigher, S.M., Simon-Rusinowitz, L., & England, S.E. (1992). *Wages for caring. Compensating family care of the elderly.* New York: Praeger.

Mahoney, K. J., Simone, K., & Simon-Rusinowitz, L. (2000). Early lessons from the Cash and Counseling Demonstration and Evaluation. *Generations, 24,* 41-46.

Mahoney, K. J., Simon-Rusinowitz, L., Loughlin, D. M, Desmond, S., & Squillace, M. (2002). Determining personal care consumers' preferences for a consumer-directed "Cash and Counseling" option: Survey results from Arkansas, Florida, New Jersey and New York elders and adults with physical disabilities. Submitted to *Health Services Research Journal*.

National Alliance for Caregiving (1997, June). Family caregiving in the U.S.: Findings from a national survey. Retrieved April 19, 2002, from *http://www.caregiving.org/finalreport.pdf*

Olmstead v. LC: 527 U.S. 581, 1999)

Sabatino, C.P. (1990). *Lessons for enhancing consumer-directed approaches in home care*. Washington, D.C. American Bar Association Commission on Legal Problems of the Elderly.

Simon-Rusinowitz, L., Mahoney, K., Benjamin, A.E. (1998). Payments to families who provide care: An option that should be available. *Generations, 22*, Fall, 69-75.

Stone, R. (1995). Forward. In R.A. Kane & K.D. Penrod (Eds.), *Family caregiving in an aging society. Policy perspectives* (pp.vii-ix). Thousand Oaks, California: Sage.

Super, N. (2002). Who will be there to care? The growing gap between caregiver supply and demand. National Health Policy Forum Background Paper, January 23, George Washington University, Washington, D.C.

Whitfield, S. & Krompholz, B. (1981). *The Family Support Demonstration Project*. State of Maryland, Office on Aging.

Wilner, M. A. (2000). Toward a stable and experienced caregiving workforce. *Generations, 24*, 60-65.

Yamada, Y. (2002). Profile of home care aides, nursing home aides, and hospital aides: Historical changes and data recommendations. *The Gerontologist, 42*, 199-206.

Zacharias, B.L. (2002). Cash and Counseling Demonstration and Evaluation. Report on Arkansas paid worker focus groups. University of Maryland, Center on Aging. College Park, MD.

Inheritance and Intergenerational Transmission of Parental Care

Richard K. Caputo

SUMMARY. This paper examines the relative influence of inheritance-related and intergenerational factors on the likelihood of adult daughters providing personal care, doing household chores, or providing income to their aging parents. The study sample (n = 399) comprises a sub-sample of the National Longitudinal Surveys, Young Women's Cohort. Findings challenge the primacy of an "ethic of care" attributed to adult children in general and adult daughters in particular in regard to filial obligation to parents when it comes to providing personal care. They also in part support "ethic of care" theories when it comes to providing financial assistance. Findings suggest that targeted legislation with specific incentives may be more effective than bully pulpit or moral exhortations to ensure sufficient care by adult children for aging baby boomers in non-institutionalized settings for as long as possible to offset the costs of more formal care in years to come. *[Article copies available for a fee from The Haworth Document Delivery Service: 1-800-HAWORTH. E-mail address: <docdelivery@haworthpress.com> Website: <http://www.HaworthPress.com> © 2005 by The Haworth Press, Inc. All rights reserved.]*

Richard K. Caputo is Professor of Social Policy and Research at Yeshiva University, Wurzweiler School of Social Work, Belfer Hall, 2495 Amsterdam Ave., New York, NY 10033-3299 (E-mail: caputo@yu.edu).

[Haworth co-indexing entry note]: "Inheritance and Intergenerational Transmission of Parental Care." Caputo, Richard K. Co-published simultaneously in *Marriage & Family Review* (The Haworth Press, Inc.) Vol. 37, No. 1/2, 2005, pp. 107-127; and: *Challenges of Aging on U.S. Families: Policy and Practice Implications* (ed: Richard K. Caputo) The Haworth Press, Inc., 2005, pp. 107-127. Single or multiple copies of this article are available for a fee from The Haworth Document Delivery Service [1-800-HAWORTH, 9:00 a.m. - 5:00 p.m. (EST). E-mail address: docdelivery@haworthpress.com].

http://www.haworthpress.com/web/MFR
© 2005 by The Haworth Press, Inc. All rights reserved.
Digital Object Identifier: 10.1300/J002v37n01_08

KEYWORDS. Adult children caregivers, ethic of care, filial responsibility, inheritances, intergenerational obligation

INTRODUCTION

This study examines the relative influence of inheritance-related and intergenerational or transmission-related factors on parental care by adult daughters. Of theoretical importance is whether adult daughters provide assistance on the basis of modeled behavior, potential gain for themselves, or social norms of filial responsibility. In regard to policy, it is important to know how parental caring and prospects of inheritance are likely to affect family support and influence the distribution of public and private transfers to aging families, especially given the likelihood that the vast majority of caregivers will continue to be women and the longstanding ambiguity surrounding the proper role of the state in promoting the primacy of family care (Bengtson, 2001; Brody, 1979; Caputo, 1999; Walker, 1996).

This study also provides additional evidence that can be brought to bear on the purportedly dispelled (Bengtson & Black, 1973) myth that "Children don't care anything about their parents except for what they can get out of them" (Shanas, 1979, p. 3). To what extent might the prospect of economic reward underlay the continuity of responsible filial behavior thought to be laid to rest two decades ago, given women's socialization to or affinity for an "ethic of care" (Caputo, 2002b; Gilligan, [1982] 1993), their generally positive attitudes toward parental care (Chatters & Taylor, 1993), and their expectations about assuming responsibility for such care (Nichols & Junk, 1997)? Women may have positive attitudes about, be favorably socialized to, and/or even morally predisposed toward the prospect of caring for their aging parents, but they may expect or hope for something tangible in return to reward their efforts, as exchange and rational choice theories would predict. The present study focuses on adult daughters because women continue to bear the brunt of kin-care responsibilities (NAC/AARP, 1997; Spitze & Logan, 1990).

LITERATURE REVIEW

The research on family support systems and older persons is fairly extensive, beginning in the 1970s and expanding quite markedly throughout the 1980s and 1990s. Much of it has been reviewed elsewhere (Caputo, 2002; Horowitz, 1985; Stum, 2000; Wolf & Soldo, 1994). What follows is a selective review of empirical studies guiding the selection of study variables.

Inheritance and Filial Responsibility

Inheritance is seen as the major mechanism used by older adults to ensure support, with kinship being its predominant conduit (Nydegger, 1983). The prospect of inheritance might account for the difference in filial responsibility reported to exist for race, with whites more likely than blacks to have higher levels (Hogan, Eggebeen, & Clogg, 1993; NAC/AARP, 1997). Wolff (2000) reports that 24.1% of white households in 1998 received an inheritance over their lifetime compared to 11.0% of black households, and the average bequest among white inheritors was $115,000 (present value in 1998) and only $32,000 among black inheritors.

Several researchers have reported on the relationships among income/wealth, inheritance, and providing care. Overall, findings are mixed, supporting both altruistic and exchange models of intergenerational filial responsibility. Cox and Rank (1992) present evidence consistent with the idea that financial transfers from parents to adult children are payments for services, whereas, as Soldo and Hill (1993) note, MacDonald's (1990) analysis of the same data provides little support for *quid pro quo* exchanges. McGarry and Schoeni (1995) report an inverse relationship between income and transfers, suggesting altruistic motivations. McGarry and Schoeni (1997), however, find no evidence that parents provide financial assistance to their children in exchange for providing care, thereby supporting altruism theory, while Henretta, Hill, Li, Soldo, and Wolf (1997) indicate that past financial transfers are good predictors of which child in a family becomes a caregiver, thereby supporting exchange theory. Kao, Hong, and Widdows (1997) report that better educated and healthier children are more likely to expect receiving an inheritance, thereby failing to support altruistic bequest theory.

In a study of pre-retirement households, Wakita, Fitzsimmons, and Liao (2000) indicate that attitudes toward intergenerational support positively affect savings net worth among whites and housing net worth among Hispanics, but negatively affect savings net worth among blacks. Silverstein, Parrott, and Bengtson (1995) report that the norm of filial obligation and anticipation of inheritance motivate sons to provide support for their parents, while daughters with weaker norms toward inheritance increase their level of support to their parents. Intergenerational affection is the factor that most motivated daughters' support for parents. In addition, previous levels of social support are positively related to daughters' support for parents.

Types of Assistance

Relying on Health and Retirement Study data, Soldo and Hill (1995) find that about 11% of married couples provide financial assistance to a parent, and about 9% spend substantial time in parent care. Among unmarried women, 10.4% provided financial assistance and 11.3% provided care. Using the same data, McGarry and Schoeni (1995) report that of respondents with at least one non-co-resident parent, 85% gave neither time nor money, 6% gave money alone, 8% gave just time, and only 1% gave both. Blacks were more likely to make financial transfers than were whites. Income/assets of the parents and number of siblings were inversely related to the probability of such transfers. Compared to married couples, widows were more likely to receive financial assistance, while single men were less likely. Eggebeen (1992) finds that blacks and Hispanics are more likely that whites to give money, while blacks are less likely than whites to provide either household or childcare assistance. Poorer health of parent increases the likelihood of providing assistance, while better health increases the likelihood of giving money.

Other Correlates of Care

Wolf and Soldo (1994) suggest that among married women caregivers are somewhat less likely to be employed than non-caregivers, but that employed caregivers work no fewer hours than those not providing parent care. These findings hold in more recent studies (e.g., Dautzenberg et al., 2000). Among black Americans, Chatters and Taylor (1993) report that married daughters are more likely than those who are separated to provide assistance and that women with more years of formal education and those who resided in rural areas tend to give help to their parents more frequently than their counterparts. This latter finding is consistent with other research showing that those raised in rural areas express stronger filial responsibility than those raised in urban areas (Lee, Coward, & Netzer, 1994).

THEORETICAL CONSIDERATIONS AND POLICY IMPLICATIONS

Following Caputo (2002a), this study distinguishes between two types of rational behaviors adult daughters exhibit in their roles as parental caregivers: rational actors vs. rational agents. Rational actors are followers of rules whose actions express a value because it is the right thing to do, while rational agents are choice makers whose actions are goal directed (Nobel, 2000). Exchange and rational choice theories provide the basis of social action in which individuals act as rational agents. They posit that people are self-interested and human behavior is best understood as an exchange of goods, material, and non-material (Coleman, 1990; Homans, 1958). To the extent adult daughters are more likely than not to be caregivers and/or income providers to parents with assets, especially when controlling for whether or not their parents were caregivers and/or income providers, they are construed as rational agents.

An exclusive focus on rational agents as participants in an exchange process focuses too narrowly on social interactions at the expense of structural determinants of human behavior (Berberoglu, 1998). In this study, rational actors are construed theoretically to follow rules or norms that have structural level properties. That is, their evolution and influence go beyond the socialization and transmission of core values within families (Bengtson, 1975; Roberts, Richards, & Bengtson, 1991). As Coleman (1990) notes, the initial properties at the structural level of exchange systems, even dyadic exchanges, are of two sorts: institutional rules or norms and distributional properties. Norms, of concern here, govern how exchanges take place. They may be minimal, such as a norm that private holdings are to be respected or that filial responsibility should be expected as a matter of course. They may be inclusive, involving how financial transactions are to be carried out or under what conditions and in what ways adult children are obligated to take responsibility for their parents. Individuals following such rules or norms are construed here as rational actors. According to Becker (1988) the influence of norms should be minimal when bequests are of concern in linking generations together.

Caputo (2002a) provided some evidence regarding how such norms influence parental assistance independently of such inheritance-related factors. Absent, however, was the role of modeling, whether or not adult daughters had the opportunity to witness their parents provide assistance to their parents' parents. If so, then adult daughters could be expected to emulate their parents' behavior, independently of other social messages about what constitutes appropriate filial responsibility. For purposes of this study, adult daughters who are caregivers and/or income providers, who believe that parents are under no obligation to leave an inheritance to their children, *and whose parents were caregivers or income providers to their parents (i.e., the adult daughters' grandparents)* are construed as rational actors.

Policy implications stem from whether adult daughters act as rational agents or actors. A major impetus for evaluating the competing models of altruism and exchange is to anticipate whether public transfers will displace private transfers, leaving recipients of public assistance at the same levels without such assistance (Cox & Rank, 1992). Motivational models based on altruism suggest that public transfer programs have no effect on the aggregate distribution of income because public transfers cancel out private transfers (Altonji, Hayashi, & Kotlikoff, 1992). Public transfer programs will have no redistributive effects if adult daughters act more like rational actors, providing care or income without expecting remuneration. Models based on exchange suggest the possibility that redistributive effects of changes in public transfers are amplified rather than cancelled. Redistributive effects of changes in public transfers may be amplified if adult daughters act more like rational agents, i.e., more consistent with the exchange theory of reciprocity. Government efforts to affect the distribution of transfers, if necessary and/or desirable, will vary accordingly. Specifically, this study addresses the extent to which adult daughters provide assistance to their parents on the basis of modeled behavior, potential gain for themselves, or social norms of filial responsibility.

METHOD

Data and Study Sample

Data came from the National Longitudinal Surveys (NLS), Young Women's Cohort, a nationally representative sample of 5,159 young women 14 to 24 years of age as of January 1, 1968. Respondents were interviewed intermittently through 1999, the most recent year of data available for this study. For the 1999 survey, 2,900 respondents were interviewed, representing 56.2% of the original sample. Documentation about the sampling and weighting procedures can be found in the *NLS Handbook 1999* (Center for Human Resource Research, 1999a).

The data are particularly suited for this study because beginning with the 1993 survey, and most extensively in 1997 and again in 1999, respondents were asked detailed series of questions about transfers of time and money to and from their parents. The study sample comprises 399 women about whom all relevant information was available and whose children were either over the age of 19, married, or parents, thereby making them eligible for time and money transfer-related questions. It should be noted that the age of these women, whose adult daughters might be providing care or financial support, ranges between 45 and 55 in 1999 and that their need for personal care and/or financial assistance might be less of a motivating factor among the adult daughters than if they had been ages 65 and older. Nonetheless, to the extent a pattern of caregiver behavior can be determined among adult daughters when their parents might be less needy by virtue of age, such a pattern is likely to carry over as parents' age and their needs increase. The same, however, cannot be said if a pattern of caregiver behavior is not found, since greater need by virtue of age may motivate adult daughters' caregiver behavior.

Measures

The families of respondents who reported that their adult children provided either personal care or did household chores for them within the preceding twelve months were classified as caregivers. The families of respondents who reported that their adult children provided financial assistance either in the form of a gift, a loan, or supplemental income to them within the preceding twelve months were classified as income providers. Following McGarry and Schoeni (1997), adult children who lived with their parents are excluded.

Table 1 identifies and defines the study variables. Of primary concern for this research is whether any of the four inheritance-related variables or either of the two transmission-related variables affect caregiver/income provider family status beyond that of other factors already known to influence these outcomes. That is, did parental assets, wills, intent to leave inheritance, expectations regarding inheritance obligations account for variation in the likelihood of respondents' children providing personal care or financial assistance to their parents when controlling for whether or not their children's grandparents had done likewise, as well as for other respondent characteristics? Several key variables warrant further elaboration.

Asset status was derived from a question asking respondents if after liquidating all assets and paying debts they would have money left over, break even, or be in debt. It was coded such that 1 = have some money left over and 0 = either owe money or break even.

TABLE 1. Definitions and Values of Study Variables

Variables	Definition/Values
Inheritance-related	
Asset status	1 = respondents with assets remaining after debts paid off, 0 = no assets remaining after debts paid off
Attitude about inheritance	1 = parents should leave an inheritance to children, 0 = parents have no further obligation to children once they leave home
Intent to leave inheritance	1 = respondents who intend to leave an inheritance to their child/children (upon their husband's death), 0 = no such intent
Will	1 = respondents who have a formal will, 0 = no will
Transmission-related	
RP financial assistance in 1997	1 = respondents provided financial assistance to their parents in 1997, 0 = provided no such assistance
RP care in 1997	1 = respondents provided personal care to or did household chores for their parents in 1997 0 = provided no such care
Respondents' Characteristics	
Age in 1999	Respondent's age in 1968 survey + 31
Education	Highest grade completed through 1999
Employment status	1 = employed at time of survey, 0 = not employed
Health status-overall	1 = fair to poor or needy, 0 = good to excellent
Health status-work related	1 = health limited ability to work, 0 = no health limitations
Low-income family	1 = family income was less than one-half the median income of the population sample, 0 = family income at or above half the median
Marital status	1 = married, 0 = other
Race	1 = Black, 0 = other, primarily White
Region	1 = South, 0 = other
Urban residency	1 = city of 50,000+ or suburb of large city, 0 = other
Respondents' Adult Children	
Caregivers	1 = provided either personal care or did household chores for their parents within the preceding twelve months, 0 = provided neither personal care nor did household chores
Income providers	1 = provided gifts, loans, or supplemental income to their parents within the preceding twelve months, 0 = provided no such financial assistance
In household	1 = presence of eligible adult children residing in the household, 0 = no eligible adult children in household

Inheritance obligation was a nominal level variable. In survey year 1997 respondents were asked to respond to the following statement: "Some people would like to leave an inheritance to their children; other people believe that once the children leave home, parents have no further obligation. How do you feel about this?" (Center for Human Resource Research, 1999b, p. 252). The variable was coded such that 1 = should leave an inheritance, and 0 = felt no further obligation. For purposes of this study, a value of 1 signified that these respondents generally felt that parents should leave an inheritance to children because this was the right thing to do.

There were two inheritance-related measures that Caputo (2002) could not use because they were unavailable in survey year 1997 which formed the basis of that study. These are whether or not the respondents had a will and their intent to leave an inheritance to their children. The former is a dichotomous measure, with 1 = having a formal will and 0 = no will. Intent to leave inheritance was a dummy variable created from two separate but related questions asked of respondents if their husbands were to die. The first question, asked of respondents with only one child, inquired if they would leave their inheritance to that child, while the second, asked of respondents with more than one child, inquired if they would leave their inheritance to those children. Respondents who intended to leave their inheritance to their child/children were coded as 1, while those indicating no such intent were coded as 0.

The transmission-related variables, RP financial assistance and RP care in 1997, were constructed from questions asked of respondents in survey year 1997 about help they gave their parents. RP financial assistance in 1997 signifies whether or not respondents reported that they provided financial assistance to their parents within the twelve months prior to the survey. RP care in 1997 signifies whether or not respondents provided personal care to or did household chores for their parents within the same period. Finally, two variables were used to capture respondents' need in regard to health. Respondents' overall health status was a dummy variable created from a question that asked respondents to compare their health to others of comparable age. A value of 1 indicated that a respondent reported her health as poor to fair compared to women of similar age, while a value of 0 indicated that she viewed her health as good to excellent compared to women of similar age. The second measure of health, also a dummy variable, captured whether or not health limited the amount or type of work that respondents could do. A value of 1 signified that health limited a respondent's ability to work, while 0 signified no such limitation.

Procedures

Logistic regression analysis is used to determine if respondents' inheritance-related factors (asset status, attitudes about inheritance, having a will, intent to leave an inheritance) or transmission-related factors (their parents' caregiver/income provider behavior) add to the explanatory power of other correlates thought to influence the likelihood of their children's caregiver/income-provider activity. Separate logistic regression procedures with the same set of correlates are used with caregiver status and income-provider status as dependent variables, with one exception in each model. To control for provision of both personal care and financial assistance, adult children's income-provider status is added to the logistic model for caregiver status, while their caregiver status is added to the model for income-provider status.

For each of the logistic regression procedures, correlates are grouped into three models. Model A (Main Effects) comprises all factors about respondents' thought to influence the likelihood of adult children's caregiver/income-provider activity, except transmission-related and inheritance-related factors. Model B (Expanded Model A) includes variables in Model A and adds the transmission-related factors. Model C (Expanded Model B) treats Model B as a Main Effects Model and adds the inheritance-related factors. The residual score statistic, Q_{RS} (Breslow & Day, 1980; Stokes, Davis, & Koch, 1995), is used to determine what if any effects the transmission-related factors had on Model A overall and the inheritance-related factors had on Model B overall, as well as on individual variables of the respective models. Ordinarily, a Main Effects Model fits adequately when the Q_{RS} statistic fails to meet statistical significance with a p-value < .05. In addition, the -2 Log Likelihood statistic is used to compare models (A vs. B, B vs. C), with lower values signifying a more desirable model (SAS Institute Inc., 1990). Finally, the Hosmer and Lemeshow Goodness-of-Fit Test is used to assess how well the data fit the Expanded Models, a good fit signified by higher p-values (Cody & Smith, 1997; Stokes, Davis, & Koch, 1995).

Limitations

As noted, the age of these women, whose adult daughters might be providing care or financial support, ranges between 45 and 55 in 1999. As a result, their need for personal care and/or financial assistance might be less of a motivating factor than if they had been ages 65 and older. The omission of affective or solidarity motivations, explored by others (e.g.,

Parrott & Bengtson, 1999; Silverstein & Bengtson, 1997) further limits this study. The study also excludes emotional and psychological dimensions that have been shown to affect inheritance decisions (Stum, 2000), as well as early family relationships and parent to child transfers of time and money that have been found to affect support provided to parents by adult children (Whitbeck, Hoyt, & Huck, 1994). By focusing on adult daughters and their parents, the study does not address the needs of those without children who would have to rely primarily on public and private mediating support services in times of need (Cantor, 1991).

RESULTS

As Table 2 indicates for respondents about whom all relevant information was available (n = 399), only four of seventeen characteristics had a bivariate relationship with the likelihood of adult daughters' providing personal care. Most significantly, women with caregiver adult daughters were five and one-half times more likely to have adult daughters who also provided financial assistance ($\chi^2 = 16.3$, p < .001) and five times as likely to have adult sons who provided personal care ($\chi^2 = 21.6$, p < .001). They were also twice as likely to have had a health condition that limited the type or amount of work they could do ($\chi^2 = 05.2$, p < .05). Finally, women with caregiver adult daughters were less likely (14.98% versus 17.7%) to be married ($\chi^2 = 03.8$, p < .05). Although none of the inheritance-related or transmission-related factors had a statistically significant relationship with the likelihood of adult daughters' providing personal care, it should be noted that women who intended to leave inheritances to their children were more than one and one-half times more likely to have daughters who provided personal care ($\chi^2 = 03.2$, p = .07).

As Table 2 also indicates, seven of seventeen characteristics had a bivariate relationship with the likelihood of adult daughters' providing financial assistance. Most significantly, women with income provider adult daughters were more than six and one-half times more likely to have adult sons who also provided financial assistance ($\chi^2 = 18.4$, p < .001) and five and one-half times more likely to have adult daughters who provided personal care ($\chi^2 = 16.3$, p < .001). They were nearly five times more likely to be black ($\chi^2 = 04.9$, p < .05). Women with income provider adult daughters were also more than three times as likely to have had a health condition that limited the type or amount of work they could do ($\chi^2 = 05.2$, p < .05) and nearly three times as likely to have poor

TABLE 2. Percentages of Women with Adult Daughter Caregivers and Income Providers Likely or Not Likely to Exhibit Study Characteristics in 1999 (n = 399)

Characteristics	Caregivers Percent		Odds/ Chi-square	Income Providers Percent		Odds/ Chi-square
	Likely	Not Likely		Likely	Not Likely	
Inheritance-related						
Assets left over	15.00	19.65	0.722/0.972	04.09	09.57	0.413/3.840*
Attitude–obligation to children	16.39	12.29	1.399/0.351	05.19	11.54	0.420/3.229
Intend to leave inheritance	19.64	13.49	1.567/3.232	03.19	06.44	0.479/1.420
Will	18.84	13.86	1.443/2.138	03.34	06.42	0.503/0.863
Transmission-related						
RP financial assistance in 1997	16.37	15.38	1.077/0.179	05.27	05.11	1.034/0.066
RP care in 1997	18.67	13.52	1.469/1.623	08.52	02.41	3.771/4.791*
Respondents						
Employed	13.90	25.69	0.467/1.816	05.02	06.03	0.823/0.224
Health status–poor to fair overall	20.60	15.12	1.457/0.505	11.20	04.14	2.847/6.161*
Health limited work	24.84	14.15	2.005/5.197*	11.55	03.97	3.157/5.216*
Low-income families	10.40	16.62	0.583/0.025	07.86	04.82	1.684/1.522
Married	14.98	17.74	0.817/3.832*	05.19	05.18	1.002/0.133
Race-Black	21.13	15.35	1.478/1.188	17.06	04.03	4.904/12.954***
Region-South	18.86	14.61	1.358/0.038	05.21	05.18	1.007/0.113
Urban residency	17.36	14.80	1.210/0.994	05.20	05.17	1.006/0.002
Respondents' Adult Children						
Daughters provided money/care[1]	47.44	14.14	5.482/16.343***	15.51	03.24	5.482/16.343***
Sons provided care/money[2]	44.87	13.96	5.017/21.553***	25.00	04.72	6.727/18.430***
Residing in home	14.91	16.19	0.906/0.205	08.92	03.91	2.408/3.612

Note: Percents are weighted based on the sampling frame in 1999. Odds ratios are based on the weighted data. Because the use of weighted data results in very large chi-squares and with statistically significant p-values, the chi-square and related p-values in the table are those of unweighted data. T-tests showed no differences between caregivers vs. non-caregivers or income providers vs. non-providers by age (49.8 years old) or years of highest grade completed (13.0).
[1] Percents of families of respondents with caregiver daughters who are likely/not to have daughters also giving financial assistance/percents with income provider daughters who are likely/not likely to have daughters also providing personal care.
[2] Percents of families of respondents with caregiver daughters who are likely/not to have sons also providing personal care/percents with income provider daughters who are likely/not likely to have sons also providing financial assistance. ***p ≤ .001; *p ≤ .05.

to fair health overall. Women respondents who had provided personal care to their parents in 1997 were more than three and one-half times more likely to be recipients of income from their own adult daughters in 1999 ($\chi^2 = 04.8$, p < .05).

Women who appeared to be more financially comfortable, i.e., they would have money left over after liquidating their assets and paying debts, were less likely to be receiving financial assistance from their adult daughters. However, only about twice as many elderly women who were not financially secure received financial help from their daughters (04.1% vs. 09.6%, $\chi^2 = 03.8$, p < .05).

Although no other inheritance-related or transmission-related factor had a statistically significant relationship with the likelihood of adult daughters' providing financial assistance, it should be noted that women who felt that parents should leave inheritances to their children were paradoxically less likely (05.2% vs.11.5%) to have daughters who provided personal care ($\chi^2 = 03.2$, p = .07).

As can be seen in Table 3, under Caregivers, Model A fit the data adequately, signifying that the transmission-related variables added no explanatory power beyond that of the other correlates. As Model B_1 indicates, neither caregiver nor income provider behavior of respondents toward their parents affected the likelihood of their adult daughters providing care. As Model B_2 indicates, the addition of the transmission-related variables to Model A did not adequately fit the data ($Q_{RS} = 11.6$, p = 0.02). As can be seen in Model C, however, the inheritance-related variable, intent to leave an inheritance to one's child or children, added to the explanatory power of Model B_2 ($Q_{RS} = 3.9$, p = 0.27). Women who intended to leave an inheritance to their children were more than two and one-half times as likely to have adult daughters as caregivers. Across all models, women whose adult daughters provided financial assistance and who also had sons as caregivers were more than five to six times as likely to have daughters as caregivers and this was most likely to occur when accounting for inheritance-related factors. In addition, married women were only about half as likely to have adult daughters as caregivers.

As can be seen in Table 3 under Income Providers, Model A did not fit the data adequately, signifying that transmission-related variables added explanatory power beyond that of the other correlates ($Q_{RS} = 6.6$, p = 0.04). In particular, as Model B_1 shows, women who provided care to or did household chores for their parents in 1997 were more than three and one-half times as likely to have adult daughters who provided

TABLE 3. Odds of Caregiver and Income Provider Activity in 1999 (n = 399)

Characteristics	Caregivers				Income Providers			
	Model A	Model B_1	Model B_2	Model C	Model A	Model B_1	Model B_2	Model C
Inheritance-related								
Assets left over				ns				ns
Attitude–obligation to children				ns				0.21*
Intend to leave inheritance				2.57**				ns
Will				ns				ns
Transmission-related								
RP financial assistance in 1997		ns		1.16		ns	0.74	0.66
RP care in 1997		ns		1.32		3.58*	3.93*	4.37*
Respondents								
Age	1.00	1.00	0.97	0.95	1.05	1.02	1.02	1.02
Education	0.98	0.98	0.99	0.97	1.06	1.01	1.02	1.03
Employed	0.54	0.54	0.55	0.55	0.76	0.94	0.91	0.81
Health status–poor to fair overall	0.79	0.79	0.80	0.78	2.45	2.77	2.80	3.25
Health limited work	1.89	1.89	1.88	1.89	1.91	1.84	1.81	1.62
Low-income families	0.54	0.54	0.54	0.53	0.72	0.45	0.43	0.41
Married	0.52*	0.52*	0.52*	0.47*	1.81	1.60	1.63	1.75
Race–Black	1.10	1.10	1.12	1.32	6.13**	7.17**	7.41**	6.77**
Region–South	1.13	1.13	1.14	1.20	0.59	0.58	0.58	0.64
Urban residency	1.12	1.12	1.09	1.04	1.01	0.88	0.92	0.87
Respondents' Adult Children								
Daughters provided money/care[1]	5.00***	5.00***	4.77**	5.28***	5.19**	4.59**	4.57**	5.48**
Sons provided care/money[2]	5.49***	5.49***	5.63***	6.76***	21.67***	31.94***	34.20***	51.16***
Residing in home	0.81	0.81	0.81	0.83	2.82*	2.64	2.61	2.92
Statistics								
Max-rescaled R^2	0.1563	0.1563	0.1594	0.1909	0.2764	0.315	0.318	0.3521
Q_{RS}	0.79, df = 2, p = 0.67	0.79, df = 2, p = 0.67	11.6, df = 4, p = 0.02	3.94, df = 3, p = 0.27	6.62, df = 2, p = 0.04	0.38, df = 1, p = 0.53	10.4, df = 4, p = 0.03	2.69, df = 3, p = 0.44
–2 Log L	316.148	316.148	315.357	307.099	138.975	132.635	132.253	126.505
Hosmer & Lemeshaw	13.2, df = 8, p = 0.11	13.2, df = 8, p = 0.11		11.1, df = 8, p = 0.19		11.9, df = 8, p = 0.16		18.2, df = 8, p = 0.02

[1]See Table 2 Note 1. [2]See Table 2 Note 2. ***p < .001; **p < .01; *p < .05.

financial assistance. As can be seen in Model B_2, however, the addition of transmission-related variables to Model A also did not fit the data adequately ($Q_{RS} = 10.4$, p = 0.03), signifying that inheritance-related factors added to the explanatory power of the model. In particular, as Model C indicates, holding the attitude that parents should leave inheritances to their children decreased the likelihood of respondents' adult daughters providing financial assistance. It should be noted in this context that women more likely to have adult daughters who provided financial assistance were also more then three times as likely to have poor to fair overall health than women of comparable age (p = .06), suggesting that health needs also play an important role in affecting the likelihood of providing financial assistance other factors being equal. Neither of the health-related variables (affecting the type/amount of work one could do or overall health) approached statistical significance (p < .10) in the caregiver models. It should also be noted that although Model C was a better model than Model B_2, signified by the lower –2 Log L statistics (126.6 vs. 132.3), the overall adequacy of Model C is questionable, denoted by the Hosmer and Lemeshaw statistics ($\chi^2 = 18.2$, p = 0.02).

Across all income provider models, women whose adult daughters provided financial assistance were more than twenty to fifty times more likely to have sons as income providers and they were nearly four and one-half to five and one-half times as likely to have daughters as caregivers. As was the case in the caregiver models, this was most likely to occur when accounting for inheritance-related factors. In addition, black women were more than six to seven times as likely to have adult daughters as income providers. Finally, even when accounting for inheritance-related factors, the transmission-related factor, respondents providing personal care to their parents in 1997, remained significant. Women caregivers in 1997 were more than four times as likely to have adult daughters who provided financial assistance.

DISCUSSION

Findings suggest that inheritance-related factors, especially intentions to leave inheritances to children, are likely to affect adult daughters' decisions to provide personal care or do household chores for their parents more than other factors accounted for in this study. Parents' caregiver behavior does not affect the likelihood of adult daughters' caregiver activity, suggesting that caregiver behavior is not modeled, i.e., transmitted from one generation to the next. As such, caregivers' behavior is consistent with rational choice or exchange theory. These findings are at variance with general social norms about filial responsibility and altruism found in recent decades to be pervasive among adult children in the United States and they challenge the primacy of the "ethic of care" attributed to adult children in general and adult daughters in particular in regard to filial obligation to parents. If exchange rather than filial responsibility continues as a major motivating factor among caregivers into the twenty-first century and thereby reverses the trends of preceding generations (Hareven, 1994), these findings pose concerns for the country as a whole for at least two reasons. First, in regard to caregiving, there may be redistributive effects of public policies that decrease the prospect or amount of inheritances that parents want to bequeath to their children. That is, excessive taxation may diminish the value of assets to such an extent that parents may lose an incentive for their adult daughters to provide personal care in times of need. Further research is needed to determine how size of anticipated inheritances might affect parents' intentions to leave inheritances as well as adult daughters' caregiver behavior. On the other hand, income received from Social Security, Medicare, Supplemental Security Income, and the like might enable parents to retain more of their assets for purposes of inheritance, thereby increasing the incentive for personal care on the part of their adult children. To the extent the cash benefits of these programs are eroded, incentives for adult children caregivers also decrease.

In regard to the second concern for the country as a whole, findings also suggest that the normative ethos is weaker than self-interest, thereby raising the possibility that, in the absence of other financial incentives, state mandated requirements may be necessary to ensure an adequate pool of caregivers in the upcoming decades as related needs of the baby boom generation increase. It may be far more effective and humane for states and/or the federal government to enable "boomer" parents to remain in their own homes and communities as long as their health permits by finding ways of remunerating their adult children who provide care or do household chores or obligating them to do so much as parents are legally obligated to care for their own pre-adult children than to underwrite institutional care or do nothing and rely solely on market forces. Reliance on the bully pulpit and moral suasion, though potentially useful, will be less effective than concrete legislative, legal policies.

This study also finds that inheritance-related factors, especially parents' attitudes about leaving inheritances to children, and transmission-related factors, especially having parents who provided care to their aging parents, affect adult daughters' decisions to provide income to their aging parents. Paradoxically, having a favorable attitude about leaving inheritances to children reduces the likelihood of having adult daughters as income providers, thereby challenging the tenets of rational choice or exchange theory and suggesting more complex motivations in regard to filial obligations. This paradox is partially accounted for by the finding that the overall health of the adult daughters' mothers also mattered, such that those in poor to fair health were also more likely to have adult daughters as income providers. It is also possible that those who had a favorable attitude towards leaving inheritances to their children might be in a more stable financial position (e.g., own a house, furniture, life insurance) to do so and therefore do not need financial help from children. To the extent adult daughters provided income to offset possible health-related expenses either directly or indirectly, these findings provide some evidence for social normative or altruistic behavior of filial responsibility based on need. Further, the finding of having parents who provided care to their aging parents provides evidence for modeled behavior of filial responsibility, thereby supporting "ethic of care" theories. These findings bode well for the nation for two reasons despite the possibility of being at odds with its caregiver needs. First, they suggest that there might be no redistributive effects of public policies that augment the income of aging parents. Income from such programs as Social Security, Medicare, Supplemental Security Income, and the like will not necessarily displace income from adult children. Second, public policies requiring parents in need to spend down their assets in return for publicly financed health benefits, for example, will not necessarily reduce the likelihood of adult children providing financial assistance. Asset reduction in excess of income from adult children, however, reduces the likelihood of adult children providing personal care to or doing household chores for their aging parents and such policies should be calibrated accordingly to reduce such possibilities or avoided.

Results and policy implications of this study should be taken cautiously in light of the previously mentioned limitations that suggest future avenues for research. In particular, intra-household transfers would be an appropriate focus of additional research, since the study accounted only for the presence of eligible adult children within the household and not for their caregiver or income provider activities. More detailed studies are also needed to document what if any deletion of personal care occurs when aging parents spend down their assets that may otherwise be used for inheritance purposes.

REFERENCES

Altonji, R.G., Hayashi, F., & Kotlikoff, L.J. (1992). Is the extended family altruistically linked? Direct tests using micro data. *American Economic Review, 82*, 1177-1198.

Becker, G.S. (1974). A theory of social interaction. *Journal of Political Economy, 82*, 1063-1093.

Becker, G.S. (1988). Family economics and macro behavior. *The American Economic Review, 78*, 1-13.

Bengtson, V.L. (1975). Generation and family effects in value socialization. *American Sociological Review, 40*, 358-371.

Bengtson, V.L. (2001). Beyond the nuclear family: The increasing importance of multigenerational bonds. *Journal of Marriage and the Family, 63*, 1-16.

Bengtson, V.L., & Black, K.D. (1973). Inter-generational relations and continuities in socialization. In P.B. Baltes & K.W. Schaie (Eds.), *Life-span developmental psychology: Personality and socialization* (pp. 207-234). New York: Academic Press.

Berberoglu, B. (1998). *An introduction to classical and contemporary social theory: A critical perspective.* 2nd ed. Dix Hills, NY: General Hall, Inc.

Boaz, R.F., & Muller, C.F. (1992). Paid work and unpaid help by caregivers of the disabled and frail elders. *Medical Care, 30*, 149-158.

Breslow, N.E., & Day, N.E. (1980). *Statistical methods in cancer research, volume I: The analysis of case studies.* Lyons, France: International Agency for Research on Cancer.

Brody, E.M. (1979). Aging parents and aging children. In P.K. Ragan (Ed.), *Aging parents* (pp. 193-207). Los Angeles: University of Southern California Press.

Cantor, M.H. (1991). Family and community: Changing roles in an aging society. *The Gerontologist, 31*, 337-346.

Caputo R.K. (2002a). Adult daughters as parental caregivers: Rational actors versus rational agents. *Journal of Family and Economic Issues, 23*, 27-50.

Caputo, R.K. (1999). Age-condensed and age-gapped families: Coresidency with elderly parents and relatives in a mature women's cohort, 1967-1995. *Marriage & Family Review, 29*, 77-95.

Caputo, R.K. (2002b). Social justice, the ethic of care, and market economies. *Families in Society, 83*, 355-364.

Center for Human Resource Research. (1999a). *NLS handbook 1999.* Columbus, OH: Ohio State University.

Center for Human Resource Research. (1999b). *NLS of mature and young women 1997 questionnaire.* Columbus, OH: Ohio State University.

Chatters, L.M., & Taylor, R.J. (1993). Intergenerational support: The provision of assistance to parents by adult children. In J.S. Jackson, L.M. Chatters, & R.J. Taylor (Eds.), *Aging in Black America* (pp. 69-83). Newbury Park, CA: Sage.

Chatters, L., Taylor, R.J., & Jackson, J.S. (1986). Aged blacks' choices for an informal helper network. *Journal of Gerontology, 41*, 94-100.

Chatters, L., Taylor, R.J., & Neighbors, H.W. (1989). Size of the informal helper network mobilized in response to serious personal problems. *Journal of Marriage and the Family, 51*, 667-676.

Cody, R.P., & Smith, J.K. (1997). *Applied statistics and the SAS programming language.* Fourth edition; Upper Saddle River, NJ: Prentice Hall.

Coleman, J.S. (1990). *Foundations of social theory.* Cambridge, MA: Belknap Press of Harvard University Press.

Connell, C.M., & Gibson, G.D. (1997). Racial, ethnic, and cultural differences in demential caregiving: Review and analysis. *The Gerontologist, 37,* 355-364.

Cox, D., & Rank, M.R. (1992). Inter-vivos transfers and intergenerational exchange. *The Review of Economics and Statistics, 74,* 305-314.

Dautzenberg, M.G.H., Diederiks, J.P.M., Philipsen, H., Stevens, F.C.J., Tan, F.E.S., & Vernooij-Dassen, M.J.F.J. (2000). The competing demands of paid work and parent care. *Research on Aging, 22,* 165-187.

Eggebeen, D.J. (1992). Family structure and intergenerational exchanges. *Research on Aging, 14,* 427-447.

Eggebeen, D.J. (1993). From, generation unto generation: Parent-child support in aging American families. In L. Burton (Ed.), *Families and aging* (pp. 91-100). Amityville, NY: Baywood Publishing Company, Inc.

Gilligan, C. ([1982] 1993). *In a different voice: Psychological theory and women's development.* Cambridge, MA: Harvard University Press.

Greenwell, L., & Bengtson, V.L. (1997). Geographic distance and contact between middle-aged children and their parents: The effects of social class over 20 years. *Journal of Gerontology: Social Sciences, 52B*(1), S13-S26.

Hareven, T.K. (1994). Aging and generational relations: A historical and life course perspective. *American Review of Sociology, 20,* 437-461.

Henretta, J.C., Hill, M.S., Li, W., Soldo, B.J., & Wolf, D.A. (1997). Selection of children to provide care: The effect of earlier parental transfers. *The Journals of Gerontology, 52B: Psychological and Social Sciences (Special Issues),* 110-119.

Hogan, D.P., Eggebeen, D.J., & Clogg, C.C. (1993). The structure of intergenerational exchanges in American families. *American Journal of Sociology, 98,* 1428-1458.

Homans, G.C. (1958). Social behavior as exchange. *American Journal of Sociology, 63,* 597-606.

Horowitz, A. (1985). Family caregiving to the frail elderly. In M.P. Lawton & G.L. Maddox (Eds.), *Annual review of gerontology and geriatrics, Volume 5* (pp. 194-246). New York: Springer Publishing Company.

Johnson C. L., & Catalano, D.J. (1981). Childless elderly and their family support. *The Gerontologist, 21,* 610-618.

Kao, Y.E., Hong, G-S., & Widdows, R. (1997). Bequest expectations: Evidence from the 1989 survey of consumer affairs. *Journal of Family and Economic Issues, 18,* 357-377.

Lee, G.R., Coward, R.T., & Netzer, J.K. (1994). Residential differences in filial responsibility expectations among older persons. *Rural Sociology, 59,* 100-109.

MacDonald, M. (1990, Spring). *Family background, the life cycle, and inter-household transfers* (Working paper). Madison, WI: University of Wisconsin, Center for Demography and Ecology.

McGarry, K., & Schoeni, R.F. (1995). Transfer behavior in the health and retirement study. *The Journal of Human Resources, 30(Supplement),* S184-S226.

McGarry, K., & Schoeni, R.F. (1997). Transfer behavior within the family: Results from the asset and health dynamics study. *The Journals of Gerontology. Series B: Psychological and Social Sciences, 52B (Special Issue),* 82-92.

NAC/AARP (1997). *Family caregiving in the U.S.: Findings from a national survey.* Bethesda, MD: National Alliance for Caregiving/Washington, DC: American Association of Retired Persons.

Nichols, L.S., & Junk, V.W. (1997). The sandwich generation: Dependency, proximity, and task assistance needs of parents. *Journal of Family and Economic Issues, 18,* 299-326.

Nobel, T. (2000). *Social theory and social change.* New York: St. Martin's Press.

Nydegger, C.N. (1983). Family ties of the aged in cross-cultural perspective. *The Gerontologist, 23,* 26-32.

Parrott, T.M., & Bengtson, V.L. (1999). The effects of earlier intergenerational affection, normative expectations, and family conflict on contemporary exchanges of help and support. *Research on Aging, 21,* 73-105.

Roberts, R.E.L., Richards, L.N., & Bengtson, V.L. (1991). Intergenerational solidarity in families: Untangling the ties that bind. *Marriage & Family Review, 16,* 11-46.

Rossi, A.S., & Rossi, P.H. (1990). *Of human bonding: Parent-child relations across the life course.* Hawthorne, NY: Aldyne de Gruyter.

SAS Institute Inc. (1990). *SAS/STAT User's Guide. Volume 2, GLM-VARCOMP.* Version 6. 4th edition; Cary, NC: Author.

Shanas, E. (1979). Social myth as hypothesis: The case of the family relations of old people. *The Gerontologist, 19,* 3-9.

Silverstein, M., Parrott, T.M., & Bengtson, V.L. (1995). Factors that predispose middle-aged sons and daughters to provide social support to older persons. *Journal of Marriage and the Family, 57,* 465-475.

Silverstein, M., & Bengtson, V.L. (1997). Intergenerational solidarity and the structure of adult child-parent relationships in American families. *American Journal of Sociology, 103,* 429-460.

Soldo, B.J., & Hill, M.S. (1993). Intergenerational transfers: Economic, demographic, and social perspectives. In G.L. Maddox & M.P. Lawton (Eds.), *Annual review of gerontology and geriatrics: Vol. 13. Focus on kinship, aging, and social change* (pp. 187-216). New York: Springer Publishing Company.

Soldo, B.J., & Hill, M.S. (1995). Family structure and transfer measures in the health and retirement study. *The Journal of Human Resources, 30(Supplement),* S108-S137.

Spitze, G., & Logan, J. (1990). Sons, daughters, and intergenerational social support. *Journal of Marriage and the Family, 52,* 420-430.

Stokes, M.E., Davis, C.S., & Koch, G.G. (1995). *Categorical data analysis using the SAS system.* Cary, NC: SAS Institute, Inc.

Stum, M.S. (2000). Families and inheritance decisions: Examining non-titled property transfers. *Journal of Family and Economic Issues, 21,* 177-202.

Wakita, S., Fitzsimmons, V.S., & Liao, T.F. (2000). Wealth: Determinants of savings net worth and housing net worth of pre-retired households. *Journal of Family and Economic Issues, 21,* 387-418.

Walker, A. (1996). The relationship between the family and the state in the care of older people. In J. Quadagno & D. Street (Eds.), *Aging for the twenty-first century: Readings in social gerontology* (pp. 269-285). New York: St. Martin's Press.

Whitbeck, L., Hoyt, D.R., & Huck, S.M. (1994). Early family relationships, intergenerational solidarity, and support provided to parents by their adult children. *Journal of Gerontology: Social Sciences, 49,* S85-S94.

Wolff, E.N. (2000). *Recent trends in wealth ownership, 1983-1998.* Working Paper No. 300. Annandale-on-Hudson, NY: The Jerome Levy Economics Institute.

Wolf, D.A., & Soldo, B.J. (1994). Married women's allocation of time to employment and care of elderly parents. *The Journal of Human Resources, 29,* 1259-1276.

Urban and Rural African American Female Caregivers' Family Reunion Participation

Letha A. Chadiha
Julie Miller-Cribbs
Jane Rafferty
Portia Adams
Robert Pierce
Swapna Kommidi

Letha A. Chadiha is Associate Professor, University of Michigan, School of Social Work. Julie Miller-Cribbs is Assistant Professor, University of South Carolina-Columbia, College of Social Work, Columbia, SC 29208 (E-mail: jmcribbs@sc.edu). Jane Rafferty is a doctoral candidate, Department of Sociology, 1225 South University, University of Michigan, Ann Arbor, MI 48109-2590 (E-mail: jraffrty@umich.edu). Portia Adams is Assistant Professor, Graduate School of Social Service, Fordham University, 113 60th Street, New York, NY 10023 (E-mail: poadams@fordham.edu). Robert Pierce is Professor Emeritus, Washington University, The George Warren Brown School of Social Work, Campus Box 1196, St. Louis, MO 63130-4899 (E-mail: billybob@gwbmail.wustl.edu). Swapna Kommidi is Community Links Manager, International Institute of Metro, St. Louis, 3654 South Grand, St. Louis, MO 63112 (E-mail: kommidis@intlinst.org).

Address correspondence to: Letha A. Chadiha, Associate Professor, University of Michigan, School of Social Work, 1080 S. University, Ann Arbor, MI 48109-1106 (E-mail: lethac@umich.edu).

This study was supported by grant R01 AG15962 from the National Institute on Aging and the Office of Research for Women's Health. Peter Dore assisted with data preparation. Mimi Lee provided technical assistance. Deborah Bybee provided statistical assistance. An earlier version of this paper was presented at the 2002 National Council on Family Relations' 64th Annual Conference.

[Haworth co-indexing entry note]: "Urban and Rural African American Female Caregivers' Family Reunion Participation." Chadiha, Letha A. et al. Co-published simultaneously in *Marriage & Family Review* (The Haworth Press, Inc.) Vol. 37, No. 1/2, 2005, pp. 129-146; and: *Challenges of Aging on U.S. Families: Policy and Practice Implications* (ed: Richard K. Caputo) The Haworth Press, Inc., 2005, pp. 129-146. Single or multiple copies of this article are available for a fee from The Haworth Document Delivery Service [1-800-HAWORTH, 9:00 a.m. - 5:00 p.m. (EST). E-mail address: docdelivery@haworthpress.com].

http://www.haworthpress.com/web/MFR
Digital Object Identifier: 10.1300/J002v37n01_09

SUMMARY. This study examined reunion participation among 256 urban and 265 rural African American female caregivers of older African Americans. A majority of caregivers reported having reunions and reported favorably about their function. Logistic regression results indicated that for urban caregivers, reporting young children, as compared to not reporting young children, and reporting two or more helpers with caregiving, as compared to reporting no other helpers, increased odds of reunion participation. Caring for an elderly person with a high number of chronic conditions decreased odds of reunion participation. For rural caregivers, higher levels of family functioning increased odds of reunion participation; being a spouse caregiver, as compared to a daughter caregiver, decreased odds of reunion participation. Post-hoc Wald chi-square test results confirmed significant urban-rural differences when predicting urban caregivers' reunion participation from two or more caregiver helpers and number of chronic conditions for the elder. Research and service implications are discussed. *[Article copies available for a fee from The Haworth Document Delivery Service: 1-800-HAWORTH. E-mail address: <docdelivery@ haworthpress.com> Website: <http://www.HaworthPress.com> © 2005 by The Haworth Press, Inc. All rights reserved.]*

KEYWORDS. African American, caregivers, family reunions, females, rural, urban

Researchers have addressed various topics on African American family life and family caregiving. Comprehensive reviews document the structure, strengths, and issues of African American families (McLoyd, Cauce, Takeuchi, & Wilson, 2002; Taylor, Chatters, Tucker, & Lewis, 1990); other literature underscores the importance of kin networks and extended family as resources for African American families (e.g., Hunter, 1997; Littlejohn-Blake & Darling, 1993). Dilworth-Anderson, Williams, and Gibson (2002), in a two-decade review on ethnic family caregiving, highlight such topics as social support, negative effects, and coping in the caregiving experience. Caregiving is the unpaid help provided typically by a daughter, spouse, other relative, or friend to an impaired or frail elderly person residing in the community (Whitlatch & Noelker, 1996).

Research on African American families and ethnic caregiving contributes much to understanding the family life and caregiving experiences of African American female caregivers. However, family reunion participation remains an unexplored topic in research on both family life and caregiving. Family reunions are important familial events in the lives of African Americans. Popular literature reports that substantial numbers of African Americans engage annually in family reunions. Almost half of African American travel and 70% of non-business travel made by African Americans is to a family reunion (Lund, 2002). Further, literature indicates family reunions serve primarily positive functions in the lives of African Americans (Auslander, 2002; Vargus, 1997a, 1997b).

Given inadequate knowledge on family reunion involvement in the context of caregiving, an exploratory study on African American female caregivers' participation in family reunions was conducted. The purpose of the study was to document caregivers' family reunion participation, clarify reunion functions, and identify familial and caregiving variables that might predict reunion participation for urban and rural caregivers. Further, the study sought to determine whether predictors of reunion participation differed significantly across the two groups of caregivers. Four research questions were addressed: (1) Do rural and urban African American female caregivers differ on reports of ever having or attending a family reunion? (2) What is the function of family reunions for caregivers? (3) Which familial and caregiving contextual variables predict family reunion participation of urban and rural female caregivers? (4) Which familial and caregiving predictors of family reunion participation show significantly different effects for urban versus rural caregivers?

Few caregiving studies have included African American rural caregivers (see Dilworth-Anderson et al., 2002). The current study is significant for including rural caregivers. It responds to a call for more research on the positive aspects of the caregiving experience (Miller & Lawton, 1997) and the family life of African Americans (Taylor, Jackson, & Chatters, 1997). Further, it fills a knowledge gap by addressing urban and rural African American caregivers' family reunion participation.

LITERATURE ON FAMILY REUNIONS AND CAREGIVING

Conceptually, family reunions are regarded as an important and positive ritual for African Americans. Fiese, Hooker, Kotary, and Schwagler (1993) have defined ritual as routine practices, organized behavior, symbols and beliefs of family's identity. Rituals provide family members with shared family identity and values; promote inter-generational communication; provide stability, organization, and conti-nuity; provide for expression of cultural or ethnic heritage, and provide family members with the strength to face experiences of oppression (Bennett, Wolin, & McAvity, 1988; Fiese, 1992; Imber-Black, 1991; Rosenthal & Marshall, 1988).

Structurally, African American family reunions are typically large affairs, last approximately two to three days, involve blood-related kin, non-blood related kin, and include food (Criswell, 2000-2004; Lund, 2002; Vargus, 1997a, 1997b). Often organized around church days, town days, or cemetery decoration days (Auslander, 2002; Criswell, 2000-2004), reunions are highly organized affairs with various events including talent shows, award ceremonies, athletic events, story telling, and workshops related to social issues such as parenting (Vargus, 1997a, 1997b).

Contemporary family reunions may play a role in the preservation of extended African American families by strengthening family ties, solid-ifying family values, and highlighting and celebrating accomplishments of young family members (Auslander, 2002; Vargus, 1997a, 1997b). An important element of African American family reunions is the inter-action that occurs between generations. Young children are offered op-portunities to talk to elders, receive advice and be provided role models. Passing important family stories from the older generation to the youn-ger generation is particularly salient to African American families with histories of slavery, oppression, and dislocation (Auslander, 2002). In conclusion, while literature on African American family reunions informs the current study, this literature lacks a systematic examination of reunions and does not focus on caregivers.

Intuitively, family reunions and caregiving can be linked through the relationships and family roles of family members. For instance, family members are the principal actors in reunions. Family members rank first among persons providing care to dependent older adults (Deimling, 1994). Further, the structure of older African Americans' caregiving network is complex, ranging from a single to multiple family caregivers and involving non-kin such as friends (Dilworth-Anderson, Williams, & Cooper, 1999a). Adult children, especially daughters, and spouses of older adults are the principal actors in the caregiving network of older African Americans (Chatters, Taylor, & Jackson, 1986; National Alli-ance for Caregiving & American Association of Retired Persons, 1997). Other blood and non-blood relatives such as siblings and daughters-in-law, respectively, also provide care to older African Americans.

Literature suggests that contextual factors such as the supportive relationships that elders have with family members, the level of physical impairment of the older adult, the caregivers' own beliefs about family caregiving, and the length of time spent in caregiving may be associated with the caregiver's functioning (Deimling, 1994; Dilworth-Anderson, Williams, & Cooper, 1999b). Further, research has established that the intergenerational caregiving role (e.g., being a grandmother) may be associated with African American female caregivers' functioning (Burton, 1996). While providing care to grandchildren may influence African American female caregivers' functioning, literature is mixed on whether that influence is adverse or not (Pruchno, 1999; Whitley, Kelley, & Sipe, 2001).

In conclusion, prior literature on caregiver functioning informs the selection of potential familial and caregiving predictor variables of caregivers' reunion participation for the current study. More concretely, familial (marital status, number of children under 18 years old, grandparent status, family functioning) and caregiving contextual variables (number of other caregiver helpers, number of elder's chronic conditions, duration of caregiving, relationship to care recipient, beliefs about caregiving) that were salient in literature and seemed to logically influence caregivers' family reunion participation were selected. Predictor variables were unaccompanied by any hypotheses, given this exploratory study.

METHODS

Sample

Data came from 521 mid-western urban (n = 256) and rural (n = 265) African American female caregivers of older African Americans, 65 years and older. Conducted between July 1999 and August 2002, this cross-sectional study focused on caregivers' social functioning, mental health, and service use. Sampling consultants of the Survey Research Center at the University of Michigan used a list of elderly African American Medicare enrollees residing in metropolitan St. Louis to generate a stratified random urban sample of elders by zip code, age, and gender. Study investigators used the urban sample of Medicare enrollees to generate a sample of urban caregivers. Because of smaller numbers, all Medicare enrollees residing in seven rural counties were used to generate the rural caregiver sample. Detailed information about the study's methodology for the rural sample can be located in Chadiha, Morrow-Howell, Proctor, Picot, Gillespie, Pandey, and Dey (in press).

Study investigators adapted the reverse screening methodology of Picot, Samonte, Tierney, and Connor (2001) to screen elders and find and recruit caregivers. This methodology required one to contact the older person, who is screened to determine his or her eligibility and the caregiver's eligibility for study inclusion. An elder was eligible for study inclusion when he or she identified as African American, Black, Negro, or Colored; was 65 years and older; received unpaid help with at least one activity in daily living (e.g., bathing, grooming, dressing) or instrumental activities in daily living (e.g., shopping, housekeeping, managing money), or decision making; and received unpaid help from an African American female. A caregiver was eligible for inclusion when she was an African American female, 18 years or older, and self-identified as the unpaid person who helped with the elder's activities in daily living, instrumental activities in daily living, or decision making.

Study staff sent letters of explanation about the study prior to contacting elders. Trained female interviewers contacted and screened elders by telephone. In the absence of telephone information for some rural elderly residents, interviewers screened elders and caregivers in their homes. After gaining written consent of caregivers, interviewers used a structured computerized questionnaire to conduct an in-home interview that lasted about two and a half hours. For in-home screening and interviewing but not for telephone screening, interviewers and participants were matched on race. Interviewers completed interviews with 521 of 592 caregivers agreeing to participate, yielding an 88% response rate. Caregivers received $15 for study participation.

Sample Characteristics

Table 1 shows that, when compared to urban caregivers, rural caregivers averaged significantly lower annual household incomes ($17,780 versus $29,531). Rural caregivers were significantly younger (Mean = 52 years versus 55 years), more likely to report children under 18 years old (37% versus 23%), and more likely to have spent more years in caregiving (Mean = 11.5 years versus 6.6 years) than urban caregivers. Median caregiving years (not shown in Table 1) are also presented, given large standard deviations relative to mean caregiving years. Median caregiving years for rural and urban caregivers were 7.0 and 5.0, respectively. Additionally, rural caregivers averaged higher scores on

TABLE 1. Caregiver Sample Characteristics by Urban and Rural

Characteristic	Urban	Rural	t, χ^2
Household income ($) (n = 226, 230)			
Mean (SD)	29531 (20237)	17780 (13440)	7.29***
Range	1500-75000	1500-75000	
Age			
Mean (SD)	55 (14.69)	52 (15.24)	2.55**
Range	21-91	19-89	
Marital status (%) (n = 254, 263)			12.24*
Married	36.61	40.68	
Divorced	21.26	11.41	
Separated	10.24	7.98	
Widowed	12.20	12.55	
Never married	19.69	27.38	
Children < 18 years old (%)	23.44	36.98	11.30***
Grandparent (%) (n = 264)	57.03	60.98	n.s.
Family functioning (n = 253, 263)			n.s.
Mean (SD)	11.2 (2.91)	11.18 (2.62)	
Range	3-15	3-15	
Duration of care			
Mean (SD)	6.56 (6.26)	11.52 (11.83)	−6.02***
Range	0-49	0-67	
Relationship to elder (%)			n.s.
Daughter	49.22	49.81	
Spouse	20.31	20.00	
Other relative	20.02	20.37	
Non-relative	10.54	9.81	
# elder's chronic conditions (n = 254)			
Mean (SD)	4.07 (1.84)	3.82 (1.99)	n.s.
Range	0-10	0-11	
Other helpers (n = 251, 263)			18.11***
None	45.02	61.22	
1 helper	21.91	20.91	
≥ 2 helpers	33.07	17.87	
Caregiving ideology (n = 252, 263)			
Mean (SD)	13.71 (4.69)	14.70 (3.87)	−2.59**
Range	3-20	2-20	

Notes: Unless otherwise noted, urban sample size is 256; rural sample size is 265. Household income is without imputed missing data. Age and duration of care are in years. Other relative includes sibling, granddaughter, niece, and daughter-in-law. Non-relatives include friends, neighbors and fictive kin.
* $p < .05$ ** $p < .01$ *** $p < .001$ n.s. = not significant

caregiving ideology (Mean = 14.7 versus 13.7) than urban caregivers. In contrast, a higher proportion of urban caregivers was divorced or separated (31% versus 19%), whereas a lower proportion of rural caregivers had never married (20% versus 27%). Urban caregivers reported a larger network of other helpers with caregiving than rural caregivers: 33% of urban caregivers reported two or more other helpers with caregiving while only 18% of rural caregivers reported the same. Urban and rural caregivers did not differ significantly on grandparent status, family functioning, relationship to elder, number of elder's chronic conditions, and gender of elder (not shown in Table 1). Approximately two thirds of care recipients were female in both samples.

Dependent Measure

The dependent variable, family reunion participation, a dichotomous variable, was measured by the question, "Has your family ever had a family reunion?" Caregivers responded spontaneously with yes or no.

Independent Measures

Familial variables. Marital status was coded as married, divorced or separated, widowed, and never married; each marital status category was coded as a dummy variable (1 = yes) with married as the reference variable. The number of children under 18 years old was derived from questions that asked: "Do you have children?" "How many?" "How old are they?" Due to positive skewness, this variable was recoded as presence of children = 1, a dummy variable. Grandparent status was assessed as "Do you have grandchildren?" and coded as 1 = yes, a dummy variable. Family functioning, a summative measure based on the work of Sherbourne and Kamberg (1992), consisted of three items that asked caregivers to rate the "amount of closeness with your family," "support you give each other," "how much you talk things over." Item responses were coded as 5 = excellent, 4 = very good, 3 = good, 2 = fair and 1 = poor. Alpha reliability coefficient was .88 for urban caregivers and .85 for rural caregivers. Scores ranged from 3-15 with scores indicating higher levels of family functioning.

Caregiving contextual variables. Duration of care was in years. Relationship to care recipient was coded as spouse, daughter, other relative (i.e., sibling, niece, granddaughter, daughter-in-law), and other non-relative (i.e., friend, neighbor, fictive kin). Each category of the relationship variable was a dummy variable with its presence coded as 1. The number of other caregiver helpers was the total number of other unpaid helpers that the caregiver reported assisted the elderly person. Because of positive skewness this variable was recoded into three categories, 0 = no other helpers, 1 = one other helper, 2 = two or more helpers. Each category of the recoded variable represented a dummy variable with its presence coded as 1. Caregiving ideology, a summative measure of traditional caregiving beliefs, was based on the work of Lawton, Kleban, Moss, Rovine, and Glicksman (1989). The measure was constructed from four items that asked about the caregiver's desire to reciprocate the care she received, giving care for the purpose of being a model for her own children, living up to family traditions, and living up to religious principles. Item responses were coded as 5 = nearly always, 4 = quite frequently, 3 = sometimes, 2 = rarely and 1 = never. Alpha reliability coefficient was .74 for urban caregivers and .67 for rural caregivers. Although the alpha for rural caregivers was slightly lower than the conventional cut off of .70, the alpha for the total sample was .71. Scores ranged between 3 and 15 with higher scores indicating higher levels of caregiving ideology.

The number of elder's chronic conditions, a measure of physical disability, was the number of times that caregivers responded "yes" to a list of 13 health problems (e.g., arthritis or rheumatism, hypertension, diabetes) that a doctor told caregivers the elderly person had. The number of chronic conditions was chosen over activities in daily living needs and instrumental activities in daily living needs because chronic conditions appeared, on face validity, to be the optimal measure of physical disability.

Control and Open-Ended Measures

Age was measured in years. Annual 1999 household income, an indicator of socioeconomic status (SES), was measured using a 22-category variable, where 1 represented none or less than $3,000, and 22 represented $75,000 or more. This categorical variable was converted to a continuous variable by assigning each caregiver the mean of the selected category. Conceptually, income appeared to be a more valid SES indicator than education when the caregiver's potential travel costs to attend reunions were considered. Thirteen percent of rural caregivers and 11% of urban caregivers were missing income data; therefore the hot deck procedure was used to impute missing data values on household income (see Little & Schenker, 1995).

Function of family reunion was an open-ended question: "What is the one most important thing your family reunion gives to you or does for you?" Two independent coders coded responses to this question that yielded categories of preserving families (i.e., statements of family interactions including reuniting members), a greater sense of belonging in families (i.e., affective statements of unity and closeness), and both preserving and belonging categories. A relatively small number of negative responses were coded as other. Statements of family preservation included: "Helps bring family and their children together," and "I get a chance to meet all the generations of my family." Examples of statements of a greater sense of belonging in families were: "We are a close family and just enjoy being with one another," and "To continue the closeness among family members." Examples of both types of these statements were: "Getting together with my family and enjoying being with one another," "It's the getting together. Gives me joy to get together because we may not see each other again." The relatively small percentage of negative or other responses included: "It makes a nervous wreck out of me because somebody isn't going to act right," and "Work you to death and hear complaints after all the hard work and effort put behind the reunion." When coders failed to reach an 80% agreement based on calculating intercoder reliability (Miles & Huberman, 1994), they discussed their differences and made another independent effort to derive categories. Coders achieved 80% intercoder agreement after two efforts.

Analysis Procedures

Chi-square analyses were conducted to examine differences on reports of ever having a family reunion. Logistic regression, the appropriate multivariate analysis for modeling a dichotomous dependent variable (DeMaris, 1995), was used to predict reunion participation from control and independent variables for urban and rural caregiver samples. Research documents caregivers' background variables are associated with caregivers' functioning (Deimling, 1994; Dilworth-Anderson et al., 2002). To rule out the potential of confounding the results of logistic regression analyses, SES and age were controlled in multivariate analyses. Results of logistic regression were presented as odds ratio and 95 percent confidence intervals. Inter-item correlations for control and independent variables were not higher than .40, thus suggesting that multicollinearity was unlikely. These analyses used the Statistical Analysis System (SAS) for Windows Version 8. Further, following the procedure outlined in Allison (1999), post-hoc analyses, including calculating Wald chi-square tests, were conducted manually to determine whether predictors that were significant for either the urban or the rural group had significantly different effects across the two groups.

RESULTS

An equal proportion of urban (83.6%) and rural (83.4%) caregivers reported ever having a family reunion; thus caregivers did not differ significantly (χ^2 = .004) by location. More than half (57.5%) of rural and almost two thirds (65.4%) of urban caregivers gave statements of preserving families. Equal proportions of rural and urban caregivers (19.0% and 19.2%, respectively) gave statements indicating reunions provide family members with a sense of belonging, whereas unequal proportions of rural and urban caregivers gave both types of responses (19.0% and 7%, respectively). A relatively small percentage of rural and urban caregivers made unfavorable comments that reflected family reunions had a negative function (4.5% and 8.4%, respectively).

Table 2 presents the results of logistic regression analyses predicting family reunion participation from familial and caregiving contextual variables for urban and rural caregivers. Different significant predictors emerged for each group when applying SES and age control variables.

For urban caregivers, those with children under 18 years old were nearly 4 times as likely to have attended a family reunion (odds ratio [OR] = 3.77; 95% confidence interval [CI] = 1.21, 13.38) compared to caregivers who reported no children under 18 years old. Urban caregivers reporting two or more helpers in the caregiving network were more than 5 times as likely to have attended a family reunion (OR = 5.68, CI = 1.98, 18.89) compared to caregivers who reported no other helper. Urban caregivers' odds of participating in family reunions decreased with each one-unit change in number of chronic conditions reported for the elderly person (OR = 0.69; CI = 0.55, 0.87). Specifically, the likelihood of urban caregivers participating in family reunions decreased by slightly more than 30% with a one-unit change in number of chronic conditions reported for the elderly person.

Two significant predictors of rural caregivers' family reunion participation emerged in multivariate results (Table 2). Higher levels of family functioning for rural caregivers were associated with an increased likelihood of participating in family reunions. The odds of rural caregivers participating in family reunions increased by almost 20% (OR =

TABLE 2. Logistic Regression Predicting Caregiver's Family Reunion Participation Controlling for Household Income and Age

Variable	Urban Odds Ratio (95% C.I.)		Rural Odds Ratio (95% C.I.)	
Household income ($)	1.00	(1.00, 1.00)	1.00	(1.00, 1.00)
Age	1.01	(0.97, 1.06)	0.97	(0.94, 1.01)
Children < 18 years old	**3.77***	(1.21,13.38)	0.92	(0.31, 2.65)
Divorced/separated	1.00	(0.27, 3.40)	0.54	(0.16, 1.76)
Widowed	0.83	(0.17, 4.01)	1.38	(0.27, 8.35)
Never married	0.66	(0.15, 2.66)	0.62	(0.17, 2.11)
Family functioning	1.00	(0.88, 1.14)	**1.19***	(1.04, 1.37)
Grandparent (% = yes)	1.88	(0.73, 4.87)	1.99	(0.82, 4.91)
Other helper = 1	1.24	(0.50, 3.27)	1.14	(0.45, 3.17)
Other helper ≥ 2	**5.68***	(1.98,18.89)	0.86	(0.33, 2.47)
# elder's chronic conditions	**0.69***	(0.55, 0.87)	1.03	(0.86, 1.23)
Duration of care	1.03	(0.97, 1.10)	1.02	(0.99, 1.06)
Spouse	1.14	(0.24, 5.37)	**0.20***	(0.05, 0.74)
Other relative	1.43	(0.47, 5.09)	0.77	(0.29, 2.12)
Non-relative	0.37	(0.12, 1.18)	0.72	(0.20, 3.14)
Caregiving ideology	0.93	(0.84, 1.01)	1.00	(0.91, 1.10)
Likelihood ratio χ^2	**37.25***		**24.91+**	
−2 log likelihood	185.51		211.14	
N	249		259	

Notes: Household income includes imputed values for missing cases. Age and duration of care are in years. Excluded category for children is no children < 18 years old; for marital status is married; for # other helpers is no other helper; for grandparent is not a grandparent; for relationship to caregiver is daughter. Confidence intervals that contain 1 are not statistically significant. Both Likelihood ratio χ^2 statistics have 16 degrees of freedom.
+ p < .10   * p < .05   ** p < .01   *** p < .001.

1.19, CI = 1.04, 1.37) for each one-unit increase in level of family functioning. Additionally, rural wife caregivers were less likely to have attended a family reunion, as compared to rural daughter caregivers. The odds of rural wife caregivers participating in family reunions decreased by 80% (OR = .20; CI = 0.05, 0.74), as compared to rural daughter caregivers.

Post-hoc results of Wald chi-square tests, comparing the urban and rural coefficients for each of the five predictors that were significant in either model, yielded two significant findings at the .01 level (Table 3). Specifically, the effects of two predictors, the presence of two or more caregiver helpers (as compared to no other helpers) and the number of chronic conditions reported for the elderly person, were significantly different across groups. Both predictors made a significant contribution to predicting reunion participation in the urban group but not in the rural group.

DISCUSSION

Consistent with largely non-empirical literature and the view that re-unions are a form of family ritual for African Americans (Criswell, 2002-2004; Fiese et al., 1993; Lund, 2002; Vargus, 1997a, 1997b), a majority of urban and rural African American female caregivers partici-pate in organized family reunions. Reunions have mostly positive func-tions for caregivers by preserving families and offering family members a sense of belonging. Further, findings underscore family reunions as an intergenerational event involving young and old family members. Functions of reunions highlight the importance of the younger genera-tion, particularly children, meeting and knowing other kin. Findings, in

TABLE 3. Results of Wald Chi-Square Statistic Comparing Significant Cross-Group Logistic Regression Beta Coefficients

	Urban		Rural			
	Beta	SE	Beta	SE	Ratio of Beta Coefficients	Wald Chi-Square for Difference
Children < 18 years	1.33*	0.60	−0.08	0.54	16.62	2.99
Family functioning	0.00	0.07	0.17*	0.07	0.02	2.81
# Other helpers ≥ 2	1.74**	0.57	−0.15	0.51	11.60	6.11**
# of elder's chronic conditions	−0.37**	0.12	0.03	0.09	12.33	7.11**
Spouse	0.13	0.79	−1.62*	0.69	0.08	2.82

Notes: Following Allison (1999), we computed ratios of urban-rural beta coefficients as a way of testing for the presence of unequal residual variation. Because ratios were not consistently above or below 1, we concluded that unequal residual variation was unlikely and used the unadjusted Wald chi-square to test for between-group differences on effects.

this regard, coincide with the view that reunions may play a vital role in preserving extended families (Vargus, 1997a, 1997b).

What selected familial and caregiving contextual variables significantly predict the family reunion participation of urban and rural caregivers? For predictors of urban caregivers' reunion participation, the presence of young children, and two or more caregivers in the elder's care network may mean that these conditions facilitate the opportunity for urban caregivers to strengthen family ties through reunion involvement. Further, the presence of young children, an indicator of caregivers' parental role, may facilitate reunion involvement of urban caregivers through the opportunity that children may offer for these caregivers' social integration in familial contexts. Pillemer, Moen, Wethington, and Glasgow (2000) argue that "social integration in a more general sociological sense [refers] to both participation in meaningful roles and the network of social contacts," which contrasts with "social isolation, or the lack of significant relationships with kin, neighbors, coworkers, and friends, and of fulfilling roles" (p. 8).

Urban caregivers are less likely to participate in family reunions when they report a high number of chronic conditions for the elder, a finding that may reflect these caregivers' concerns about traveling long distances with a physically disabled elder. Further, this finding may also reflect caregivers' safety and security concerns about leaving an elder alone or in someone else's care. Irrespective of reason for the concern, failure to participate in reunions may limit opportunity for a caregiver of a physically disabled elder to benefit from the positive aspects of family reunions such as re-establishing and strengthening extended family ties (Vargas, 1997a, 1997b).

Higher levels of family functioning for rural caregivers increases reunion participation, a finding that may reflect on these caregivers' motivation to attend family reunions in order to sustain and nurture ongoing family relationships. Family functioning measures the extent to which caregivers share, support, and feel close to other family members. That rural wife caregivers, as compared to rural daughter caregivers, are less likely to participate in family reunions may mean wives are more involved in the role of family caregiving and less connected to other family life domains. Prior research documents that wives especially are vulnerable to isolation because of greater involvement in the caregiving role (see Hoyert & Seltzer, 1992).

This study may be unique in reporting significant urban-rural differences when predicting urban caregivers' reunion participation from the elder's disability status and two or more multiple helpers as compared to no other helpers. Findings are consistent with literature that documents the elderly person's level of impairment and supportive relationships with other people, especially family members, are associated with caregiver functioning (Deimling, 1994; Dilworth-Anderson et al., 2002). Further, the multiple helper finding corroborates the claim of Dilworth-Anderson et al., that "ethnic minority families usually give care in an extended family system where it is likely that multiple caregivers, and not just a primary caregiver, play central roles in providing care to dependent elders" (p. 267).

The findings from this study must be considered in light of limitations. Multivariate findings are associations and not causal. Frequency of reunion attendance would have provided a more precise measure than the dichotomous variable, ever having a family reunion. Study findings may not generalize to African American female caregivers living in other geographical areas, male caregivers of the same race, or caregivers of a different ethnic or racial group. Caregiver reports do not include the perspectives of the multiple helpers in the caregiving network of the elderly person, which may not coincide with this study's results.

Despite the limitations, this study has numerous strengths. Reunion participation highlights a positive aspect of the caregiver's family life. The study provides data on a relatively large, systematic sample of rural and urban caregivers. Significant predictors of caregivers' reunion participation emerge from both familial and caregiving contextual variables independent of age and SES that may have accounted for that participation. Post-hoc analyses establish significant urban-rural differences when predicting urban caregivers' reunion participation.

IMPLICATIONS FOR RESEARCH AND SERVICE DELIVERY

Family reunions and caregiving are dynamic events, thus suggesting a longitudinal research design might capture fuller meaning of both process and function in research on these events. Results suggest that it is important to consider both familial and caregiving variables in future studies when predicting reunion participation of urban and rural African American female caregivers. Future research should also consider other predictor variables (e.g., intergenerational interactions between young and old) that were not examined but suggested in reunion literature. Results confirming significant urban-rural differences on the predictive effects of elder's disability status and multiple caregiving help among urban caregivers suggest the need to examine heterogeneity among African American female caregivers. In this regard, future research might benefit from using larger and more heterogeneous samples. Findings should be replicated on additional samples of African American female caregivers in order to reach firmer conclusions, given this was an exploratory study.

Walker, Pratt, and Eddy (1995) note that "the formal system has unique and vital resources–particularly expertise and power–and the informal network has equally vital and unique resources–particularly proximity, affection, long-term commitment, and intense knowledge of the elder" (p. 409). Viewed in this way, service providers may want to build partnerships with African American female caregivers to help maximize resources that facilitate reunion attendance. That caregivers report mostly positive functions from involvement in family reunions implies formal resources that promote short-term relief from caregiving. Significant within-group predictors of reunion participation suggest service providers should consider both familial and caregiving contextual variables when developing services. Urban-rural differences on the significant effects of the elder's disability status and multiple caregiving help for urban caregivers' reunion participation suggest service providers cannot assume African American female caregivers are a homogenous group on the basis of same race. Rather a contextual approach may be more appropriate when developing services that promote reunion involvement. Further, significant urban-rural differences suggest that respite services may promote involvement in reunion participation among urban caregivers of disabled elders. For instance, respite services that insure an urban disabled elder is safe and secure may facilitate the urban caregiver's reunion involvement, when she fears leaving the elder alone or in someone else's care. That two or more helpers in the caregiving network increases reunion participation among urban caregivers suggests services that help mobilize the informal network.

In conclusion, the vitality of family reunions as sources of support to African American female caregivers must be carefully considered by service providers. Research that documents such support may lead to more nuanced approaches to research and service delivery. Study findings provide critical baseline information on urban and rural caregivers' family reunion participation in the context of caregiving. Much can still be learned about family reunions and caregiving. This study's findings will hopefully motivate more research on this topic.

REFERENCES

Allison, P.D. (1999). Comparing logit and probit coefficients across groups. *Sociological Methods and Research, 28,* 186-208.

Auslander, M. (2002, April). Something we need to get back to: Mythologies of origin and rituals of solidarity in African American working families. (Working Paper No. 6). Atlanta, GA: The Emory Center for Myth and Ritual in American Life.

Bennett, L.A., Wolin, S.J., & McAvity, K.J. (1988). Family identity, ritual, and myth: A cultural perspective on life cycle transitions. In C.J. Falicov (Ed.), *Family transitions* (pp. 211-234). New York: Guilford Press.

Burton, L.M. (1996). Age norms, the timing of family roles transitions, and intergenerational caregiving among African-American women. *The Gerontologist, 36,* 199-208.

Chadiha, L.A., Morrow-Howell, N., Proctor, E.K., Picot, S.J., Gillespie, D.C., Pandey, P., & Dey, A. (in press). Involving rural older African Americans and their female informal caregivers in research. *Journal of Aging and Health.*

Chatters, L.M., Taylor, R.J., & Jackson, J.S. (1986). Aged blacks' choice for an informal helper network. *Journal of Gerontology, 41*(1), 94-100.

Criswell, S. (2000-2004). Why I study family reunions. *Drylongso.* Retrieved February 27, 2002, from http://www.drylongso.com/series/genealogy/neh-1.html

Deimling, G.T. (1994). Caregiver functioning. *Annual Review of Gerontology and Geriatrics, 14,* 257-280.

DeMaris, A. (1995). A tutorial in logistic regression. *Journal of Marriage and the Family, 57,* 956-968.

Dilworth-Anderson, P., Williams, S., & Cooper, T. (1999a). Family caregiving to elderly African Americans: Caregiver types and structures. *Journal of Gerontology: Social Sciences, 54B,* S237-S241.

Dilworth-Anderson, P., Williams, S., & Cooper, T. (1999b). The contexts of experiencing emotional distress among family caregiving to elderly African Americans. *Family Relations, 48,* 391-396.

Dilworth-Anderson, P., Williams, W.S., & Gibson, B.E. (2002). Issues of race, ethnicity, and culture in caregiving research: A 20-year review (1980-2000). *The Gerontologist, 42,* 237-272.

Fiese, B.H. (1992). Dimensions of family rituals across two generations: Relation to adolescent identity. *Family Process, 31,* 151-162.

Fiese, B.H., Hooker, K.A., Kotary, L., & Schwagler, J. (1993). Family rituals in the early stage of parenthood. *Journal of Marriage and the Family, 55,* 633-642.

Hoyert, D.L., & Seltzer, M. (1992). Factors related to the well-being and life activities of family caregivers. *Family Relations, 41,* 74-81.

Hunter, A.G. (1997). Counting on grandmothers: Black mothers' and fathers' reliance on grandmothers for parenting support. *Journal of Family Issues, 18,* 252-269.

Imber-Black, E. (1991). Rituals and the healing process. In F. Walsh & M. McGoldrick (Eds.), *Living beyond loss: Death in the family* (pp. 207-223). New York: W.W. Norton.

Lawton, M. P., Kleban, M.H., Moss, M., Rovine, M., & Glicksman, A. (1989). Measuring caregiving appraisal. *Journal of Gerontology: Psychological Sciences, 44,* P61-71.

Little, R., & Schenker, N. (1995). Missing data. In G. Arminger, C. Clogg & M.E. Sobel (Eds.), *Handbook of statistical modeling for the social and behavioral sciences* (pp. 39-75). New York: Plenum Press.

Littlejohn-Blake, S., & Darling, C. (1993). Understanding the strengths of African American families. *Journal of Black Studies, 23*, 460-471.

Lund, E. (2002, August 21). Family reunions are more popular than ever [Electronic Version]. *Christian Science Monitor*, p. 11. Retrieved November 13, 2002, from http://www.csmonitor.com/2002/0821/p11s02-lifp.html

McLoyd, V.C., Cauce, A.M., Takeuchi, D., & Wilson, L. (2002). Marital processes and parental socialization in families of color: A decade review of research. *Journal of Marriage and the Family, 62*, 1070-1093.

Miles, M.B., & Huberman, A.B. (1994). *Qualitative data analysis*. Thousand Oaks: Sage Publications.

Miller, B., & Lawton, M.P. (1997). Introduction: Finding balance in caregiver research. *The Gerontologist, 37*, 216-217.

National Alliance for Caregiving & American Association of Retired Persons (1997). *Family caregiving in the U.S.: Findings from a National Survey*. Bethesda, MD: National for Caregiving. Washington, DC: AARP.

Picot, S.F., Samonte, J., Tierney, J.A., & Connor, J. (2001). Effective sampling of rare population elements: Black female caregivers and noncaregivers. *Research on Aging, 23*, 694-712.

Pillemer, K., Moen, P., Wethington, E., & Glasgow, N. (2000). Introduction. In K. Pillemer, P. Moen, E. Wethington, & N. Glasgow (Eds.), *Social integration in the second half of life* (pp. 19-47). Baltimore: Johns Hopkins University Press.

Pruchno, R. (1999). Raising grandchildren: The experiences of Black and White grandmothers. *The Gerontologist, 39*, 209-221.

Rosenthal, C.J., & Marshall, V.W. (1988). Generational transmission of family ritual. *American Behavioral Scientist, 31*, 669-684.

Sherbourne, C.D., & Kamberg, J. (1992). Social functioning: Family and marital functioning measures. In A.L. Stewart and J.E. Ware, Jr. (Eds.), *Measuring functioning and well-being* (pp. 182-193). Durham: Duke University.

Taylor, R.J., Chatters, L.M., Tucker, M.B., & Lewis, E. (1990). Black families. *Journal of Marriage and the Family, 52*, 993-1014.

Taylor, R.J., Jackson, J.S., & Chatters, L.M. (1997). Introduction. In R.J. Taylor, J.S. Jackson and L.M. Chatters (Eds.), *Family life in Black America* (pp. 1-13). Thousand Oaks, CA: Sage Publications.

Vargus, I. (1997a). Family reunions–More than a picnic–A gathering of generations. *Pathfinders Travel Magazine, Summer/Fall*.

Vargus, I. (1997b). Organizing a family reunion. *Pathfinders Travel Magazine, Summer/Fall*.

Walker, A.J., Pratt, C.C., & Eddy, L. (1995). Informal caregiving to aging family members: A critical review. *Family Relations, 44*, 402-411.

Whitlatch, C.J., & Noelker, L.S. (1996). Caregiving and caring. In J.E. Birren (Ed.), *Encyclopedia of gerontology, 1*, 253-268. San Diego, CA: Academic Press.

Whitley, D.M., Kelley, S.J., & Sipe, T.A. (2001). Grandmothers raising grandchildren: Are they at increased risk of health problems? *Health and Social Work, 26*, 105-114.

Grandparents Raising Their Grandchildren

Bert Hayslip, Jr.
Patricia L. Kaminski

SUMMARY. Grandparents who raise their grandchildren have become more prevalent as an alternate family form that is, by its very nature, intergenerational in character. This paper explores the state of our knowledge about such grandparents in light of the following themes: (1) the diversity among grandparent caregivers, (2) the importance of social support for such persons and the impact of raising a grandchild on relationships with others, (3) theoretical perspectives on grandparents raising their grandchildren, (4) the salience of issues related to parenting among grandparent caregivers, and (5) interventions with custodial grandparents. The implications of these issues for current and future cohorts of grandparent caregivers are discussed, as are directions that future work with such grandparents might take in light of these issues. *[Article copies available for a fee from The Haworth Document Delivery Service: 1-800-HAWORTH. E-mail address: <docdelivery@haworthpress.com> Website: <http://www.Haworth Press.com> © 2005 by The Haworth Press, Inc. All rights reserved.]*

Bert Hayslip, Jr. is Regents Professor of Psychology, Department of Psychology, University of North Texas. Patricia L. Kaminski is Assistant Professor of Psychology, Department of Psychology, P.O. Box 311280, University of North Texas, Denton, TX 76203-1280 (E-mail: kaminskip@unt.edu).

Address correspondence to: Bert Hayslip, Jr., Department of Psychology, P.O. Box 311280, University of North Texas, Denton, TX 76203-1280 (E-mail: hayslipb@unt.edu).

[Haworth co-indexing entry note]: "Grandparents Raising Their Grandchildren." Hayslip, Jr., Bert, and Patricia L. Kaminski. Co-published simultaneously in *Marriage & Family Review* (The Haworth Press, Inc.) Vol. 37, No. 1/2, 2005, pp. 147-169; and: *Challenges of Aging on U.S. Families: Policy and Practice Implications* (ed: Richard K. Caputo) The Haworth Press, Inc., 2005, pp. 147-169. Single or multiple copies of this article are available for a fee from The Haworth Document Delivery Service [1-800-HAWORTH, 9:00 a.m. - 5:00 p.m. (EST). E-mail address: docdelivery@haworthpress.com].

http://www.haworthpress.com/web/MFR
© 2005 by The Haworth Press, Inc. All rights reserved.
Digital Object Identifier: 10.1300/J002v37n01_10

KEYWORDS. Grandparenting, custodial grandparenting, surrogate parents, skipped-generation families, nontraditional grandparents

Custodial grandparenting is a growing trend in American society today. In 1997, approximately 5.5 million grandparents reported housing their own grandchildren (Casper & Bryson, 1998), with more recent figures in this respect increasing slightly (5.7 million) (Bryson, 2001). While most such grandparents are between the ages of 55 and 64, nearly 20% are over the age of 65 (U.S. Bureau of the Census, 2003). Regarding grandchildren, there has been a 30% increase since 1990 in the numbers of children (half of whom are under the age of 6) living in grandparent-headed households (U.S. Bureau of the Census, 2003). Of all American children in the late 1990s, 6% were living in households maintained by grandparents (Fuller-Thomson & Minkler, 2001). Recent census data (U.S. Bureau of the Census, 2003) suggest this figure to have increased slightly (6.3%), representing nearly 4.5 million children, for whom poverty is a daily problem with which they must cope. Moreover, grandchildren may also lack benefits under a custodial grandparent's insurance and have difficulty in registering for school (Ehrle, 2001; Kirby & Kaneda, 2002; Silverstein & Vehvilainen, 2000).

As both public interest and research speaking to the phenomenon of grandparents who raise their grandchildren has grown exponentially over the last decade, there is no shortage of information regarding the challenges to one's way of life, future goals, health, and well-being that raising a grandchild brings to grandparents who are often in their 50s and 60s. Those domains which seem to be most affected by custodial grandparenting reflect physical and mental health, role-specific responsibilities (e.g., role overload, role confusion), relationships with age peers (social isolation), relationships with those grandchildren one is and is not caring for, and parenting for the second time (see Cox, 2000a; Emick & Hayslip, 1999; Jendrek, 1994; Minkler & Roe, 1993; Hayslip, Shore, Henderson, & Lambert, 1998; Shore & Hayslip, 1994). In particular, many authors (see Burton, 1992; Kelley, Whitley, Sipe, & Yorker, 2000) have documented higher rates of depression and psychological distress among custodial grandparents (grandmothers) versus noncustodial grandmothers (see Fuller-Thomson & Minkler, 2000; Minkler, Fuller-Thomson, Miller, & Driver, 1997; Pruchno & McKinney, 2000). This difference is underscored by feelings of entrapment and resentment at having a dysfunctional adult child, and the presence of health problems serious enough to jeopardize custodial grandparents' ability to parent

(Kelley, 2003). In this light, grandmothers raising grandchildren are more likely to report limitations in performing daily activities of living (Minkler & Fuller-Thomson, 2001). While many such persons persevere in carrying out their responsibilities in spite of any physical limitations or symptoms, they rarely seek help for themselves, heightening their vulnerability (Hayslip & Shore, 2000).

Despite the fact that custodial grandparenting has been termed a life "countertransition," dependent upon the actions of others (Hagestad, 1988), most custodial grandparents believe they would still choose to take responsibility for their grandchildren (Hayslip et al., 1998). However, they often feel as if they are alone in this situation, and the everyday tasks associated with child rearing prevent them from engaging in activities they once enjoyed or the plans they envisioned for themselves at this stage in their lives (Jendrek, 1994). Their caretaking responsibilities often take the time once reserved for their noncustodial grandchildren, which creates guilt when they cannot spend quality time with these other grandchildren (Emick & Hayslip, 1996). Furthermore, some grandparents believe that their relationship with their custodial grandchild deteriorates after entering this parenting role (Hayslip et al., 1998). Many custodial grandparents also experience grief over the various losses that have placed them in the caregiving role (Pinson-Millburn, Fabian, Schlossberg, & Pyle, 1996). They often grieve over the loss of their own child when the adult child has died, is incarcerated, or has simply neglected to care for the child effectively (Baird, 2003). Furthermore, they fear for their grandchildren's well-being should they become unable to provide care due to physical or mental incapacitation, or if they should die (Shore & Hayslip, 1994). These consequences are even more severe when the grandchild displays problems such as hyperactivity, learning difficulties, resistance to authority, and depression (Emick & Hayslip, 1999; Hayslip et al., 1998; Hayslip & Shore, 2000) or when the parents have abused drugs (Hirshorn, Van Meter, & Brown, 2000).

While much of the literature has emphasized the negative impact of this role on middle-aged and older persons, it is important to stress that there are advantages to raising one's grandchild as well. For example, grandmothers report that the caregiving role affords them a second chance at successful parenting (Ehrle & Day, 1994; Gatti & Musatti, 1999); they can improve upon previous parenting behaviors that they now deem negative. Being a caregiving grandparent can be rewarding in and of itself, and in this light, only 19% of custodial grandparents in one study rated caregiving as "mostly stressful" (vs. rewarding)

(Giarrusso, Silverstein, & Feng, 2000). Grandparents also receive plea-sure from their especially close relationship with the grandchild whom they parent (Ehrle & Day) and feel more useful and productive as indi-viduals (Emick & Hayslip, 1999).

This paper examines the current state of our knowledge about middle aged and older persons who are raising their grandchildren on a full-time basis, termed "custodial grandparents" (Shore & Hayslip, 1994). In so doing, our discussion is organized around several salient is-sues that have come to define the study of custodial grandparents which have implications for both researchers and practitioners: (1) theoretical and conceptual frameworks relevant to the study of custodial grandpar-ents, (2) diversity among grandparent caregivers, (3) the importance of social support in the lives of such grandparents, (4) the impact of caregiving on relationships with others, (5) the salience of acquiring parenting skills for such grandparents, and (6) the availability and effi-cacy of helping interventions for grandparent caregivers.

THEORETICAL PERSPECTIVES ON CUSTODIAL GRANDPARENTING

In spite of the increase in research focusing on grandparents raising grandchildren, there has been little work in the development of theory that might guide such work. Perhaps most importantly from a lifespan perspective (see Baltes, 1997), framing custodial grandparenting in light of both its antecedents and consequences is a perspective that is most fruitful (Hayslip & Patrick, 2003). As grandparents often assume caregiving under adverse and often unpredictable circumstances and may be motivated to perform their newly acquired roles by a variety of concerns, attention to the multiple sociocultural, interpersonal, and intrapersonal antecedents of grandparent caregiving as well as to the multidimensional nature of such outcomes seems warranted.

Studying grandchildren's perceptions of their grandparents as well as those of their grandparents in anticipation of their new roles (see Somary & Stricker, 1998) can further aid in the identification of the multiple antecedents and consequences of grandparent caregiving. Greater emphasis on the dynamic nature of grandparent-grandchild re-lationships as well as more attention to cohort differences in custodial grandparenting (to include changes in the meaning of grandparenting) is warranted by existing data (see Hayslip, Henderson, & Shore, 2003; Uhlenberg & Kirby, 1998). Changes in longevity and life expectancy as well as changing expectations of the roles grandparents are expected to fill will create new cohorts of grandparent caregivers (see Uhlenberg & Kirby, 1998). In light of the historical shifts in the nature of grandparenting that have been discussed by Uhlenberg and Kirby, such changes are no less likely to impact grandparents raising their grandchildren. Likewise, attention to the construct of levels of intervention (Danish, 1981) as well as to the proximal and distal effects of any programmatic intervention is important in its design and implementation. Last, a more accurate picture of custodial grandparenting can be painted via attention to the societal context in which middle aged and older persons raise their grandchildren. Distinguishing between relationships with one's custodial and noncustodial grandchildren, spouse, service providers, and adult child might be valuable in this regard.

With regard to the distinctions between age graded, history graded, and nonnormative causes of change (Baltes, 1997), custodial grandparenting can be construed in biological terms, as when one argues that illness or death might affect one's relationship with grandchildren and possibly undermine one's ability to provide care (Solomon & Marx, 1995). Alternatively, viewing grandparent caregiving in sociocultural terms reflects the fact that changes in the incidence of divorce, or sociodemographic shifts in the nature of caregiving have literally created the phenomenon of custodial grandparenting (Uhlenberg & Kirby, 1998). Increases in deaths due to AIDS or Alzheimer's disease, elder abuse, or child abuse will further change the grandparent caregivers of the future (Joslin, 2002). New family forms will therefore emerge in light of the changing nature of grandparenting to the extent that the stigma of being a custodial grandparent may lessen. This is significant in that relative to the traditional grandparent role, grandparent caregivers often report isolation from age peers and a lack of social support (see above). This interpersonal dimension of the experience of being different from one's age peers deserves more attention than it has received thus far in the custodial grandparenting literature.

It is instructive to explore the diverse nature of theory-driven processes that might impact the adjustment of grandparents who are raising their grandchildren. For example, one might predict on the basis of Role Theory as discussed by Burnette (1999b) that roles that are unanticipated and/or ambiguous, i.e., custodial grandparent caregiver, might require more social resources so that individuals might cope with their demands. In this light, what often complicates custodial grandparenting is that grandparents have typically previously endorsed the norm of noninterference, wherein mothers emphasize the utility of grandparents' practical and moral support in child rearing, while concurrently expecting grandparents to avoid interfering in the upbringing of their grandchildren (Thomas, 1990). As a result, grandparents are often reluctant to interfere, only doing so when a crisis develops. As reliable social support can provide many health-related and psychosocial benefits to older adults (Unger, McAvay, Bruce, Berman, & Seeman, 1999), workable social convoys of support (Antonucci, 1990; Kahn & Antonucci, 1980) may permit some grandparents to adapt to their surrogate parental roles. Also crucial to this process is the identification of critical significant others under stressful circumstances via a process of socioemotional selectivity (Carstensen, 1995), as well as an accurate assessment of both role demands and one's own resources to deal with the requirements of grandparental caregiving (see Pearlin, Mullan, Semple, & Skaff, 1990). Attachment theory (Ainsworth, 1989) might also prove a fruitful avenue by which to frame variations in adjustment to this newly defined family system, viewed from both the grandparent's as well as the grandchild's perspective. Likewise, theoretical developments in the psychology of grief and loss might also hold keys to understanding grandparents' ambivalence, guilt, or hostility directed to the adult parent whose child is being raised by the grandparent, or to the grandchild's relationship to the parent who has abandoned him/her (Hayslip & Shore, 2000). For example, the Stroebe and Schut (1999) dual process model of grief, i.e., thinking about grief in both loss-oriented and restoration-oriented terms, is consistent with a multi-leveled approach to coping with loss, and might be utilized in this regard. Indeed, one might argue that grief and loss are the most salient underlying issues experienced by grandparent caregivers (Baird, 2003).

DIVERSITY AMONG GRANDPARENT CAREGIVERS

Given the heterogeneity among older adults in general (Nelson & Dannefer, 1992), it should come as no surprise that despite the many commonalities defining grandparents raising grandchildren, diversity is their outstanding characteristic. The majority of custodial grandparents are female, married, and reside in the Southern U.S. (Fuller-Thomson & Minkler, 2000; U.S. Bureau of the Census, 2003). While fifty-six percent hold jobs, 19% maintain incomes in the poverty range, and most are under the age of 65 (U.S. Bureau of the Census, 2000). Although annual incomes of these grandparents vary, in general, they are below those of traditional, noncaregiving grandparents (Fuller-Thomson &

Minkler, 2001). These figures implicitly suggest that while such persons certainly exist, we know relatively little about male custodial grandparents, about those who are widowed or divorced, raising their grandchild alone, older grandparents, or about custodial grandparents in rural areas (see Robinson, Kropf, & Myers, 2000).

The circumstances under which grandparents find themselves in the caregiving role vary as well, contributing to their heterogeneity. Divorce, adult parent drug abuse, and child abuse appear to be most common (Emick & Hayslip, 1999; Hayslip et al., 1998), but teen pregnancy, incarcerated parents, and mental or physical impairment or death of a parent can also thrust grandparents into this new role. Moreover, grandparents who provide primary care to their grandchildren do so for differing reasons. Many do not want to see their grandchildren placed in foster homes, while others perceive themselves as the only ones who are available to raise a child. Some desire to nurture their grandchildren, believe that they can provide better care than the parent, or both. Others simply offer to care for their grandchildren in order to help their own adult children in times of crisis (Hayslip et al., 1998). Grandparents also differ regarding the extent of care they provide, ranging from those who provide care occasionally and/or on a part-time basis, those who essentially provide day care only, to those who provide full-time care, to those who provide extensive secondary care (Fuller-Thomson & Minkler, 2001). In some cases, adult children may co-reside with such grandchildren and assist in their care, while others visit their children periodically, dropping in and out of their lives, often with disastrous emotional consequences for the child (Hirshorn et al., 2000; Wohl, Lahner, & Jooste, 2003). The most rapidly increasing living arrangement however, involves "skipped generation" family units, where grandchildren and grandparents live together with neither parent present (Casper & Bryson, 1998; Fuller-Thomson & Minkler, 2001).

While many parameters differentiate grandparents raising grandchildren, ethnicity/race and gender have emerged as the most important. In this respect, most grandparent caregivers are female (see Hayslip & Patrick, 2003), and most custodial grandparents categorize themselves as Caucasian (62%), African American (27%), or Hispanic (10%) (Fuller-Thomson & Minkler, 2001). Pruchno (1999) found White and Black grandmothers to differ with regard to marital status, work status, income, and household composition; Black grandmothers were more likely to have peers living with them, to have come from families with multiple generations living together, and to be getting more formal social service support. Among African American families, grandmothers are seen as buffers against the detrimental effects of an insensitive mother, and grandfathers serve as role models for boys who do not often see their fathers (Burton & DeVries, 1993; Minkler, Roe, & Robertson-Beckley, 1994). Indeed, stress and coping models of adjustment have been developed especially for African American grandparent caregivers (Crowther & Rodriguez, 2003), reflecting their unique needs.

There is also some limited work on Hispanic and/or Latino populations (Burnette, 1999a, 1999b, & 2000), examining both physical and mental health, social support, and life stress parameters defining such persons. In this respect, Goodman and Silverstein (2002) found that well-being interacted with ethnicity (Black, White, Latino), dependent upon whether grandparents were raising children without their child's assistance, or upon whether they "coparented" with the adult child. Moreover, Cox (2000b) has found Latino grandparents to be more likely to co-parent, consistent with an emphasis on the family as an on-going entity (see Cox, Brooks, & Valcarcel, 2000). Toledo, Hayslip, Emick, Toledo, and Henderson (2000) found a similar emphasis on maintaining the family to differentiate United States and Mexican custodial grandparents. Ethnic differences between European and U.S. born African American grandparent caregivers have also been found (Harper & Hardesty, 2001).

Recent work by the first author also suggests that there exists two distinct groups of custodial grandparents: (1) those whose difficulties primarily deal with the new demands of the parenting role and (2) those whose difficulties primarily revolve around having to raise a problem grandchild (Emick & Hayslip, 1999; Hayslip et al., 1998). Each group of surrogate parents faces unique sets of difficulties that may undermine their personal, marital, social, and role adjustment. Likewise, children with developmental disabilities (McKinney, McGrew, & Nelson, 2003; Kolomer, McCallion, & Overeynder, 2003) are unique, as are those who are HIV+ (Joslin, 2000, 2002), and are quite variable in terms of the desired focus of a support group intervention (Kolomer et al., 2003). The diversity among grandparent caregivers highlights the need for mental health professionals to gather personal histories from the custodial grandparents with whom they work in order to understand their unique circumstances and to best meet their needs (Wohl et al., 2003). This diversity also underscores the error in overgeneralizing about grandparents who raise their grandchildren (Hayslip & Patrick, 2003).

THE IMPORTANCE OF SOCIAL SUPPORT FOR CUSTODIAL GRANDPARENTS

In general, studies of custodial grandparents have identified social isolation and inadequate social support networks as key problems. Deficiencies include lack of emotional support (e.g., friendships, empathy) as well as tangible support (e.g., respite, child care) (Burton, 1992; Ehrle, 2001; Minkler & Roe, 1993), each compared to the availability of social support for noncustodial grandparents who provide supplemental child care (Musil, 1998). Given the critical role of social support in coping with stress (Thoits, 1995), it is clear that custodial grandparents are at risk for high levels of stress and the problems that accompany it. For example, greater perceived emotional and tangible support is associated with less depression (Musil, 1998), and lessens the negative effect of stress on self-esteem among custodial grandparents (Giarrusso, Silverstein, & Feng, 2000). Rural custodial grandparents (Robinson, Kropf, & Myers, 2000) and those raising grandchildren with emotional, behavioral, or learning problems (Emick & Hayslip, 1999) are particularly at risk for inadequate social support, and moreover, may not have access to social services, in contrast to their urban, problem-free, counterparts.

What accounts for this lack of support from others? Indeed, given the tremendous effort necessary to raise a child, the isolation of custodial grandparents appears to be directly related, at least in part, to the demands of the parenting role (see below). For example, nearly 40% of grandparent caregivers in one study attributed their isolation from friends to parenting responsibilities (Shore & Hayslip, 1994). In this light, in addition to receiving fewer social invitations, custodial grandparents decline invitations because their young charges are not welcome or they cannot afford a babysitter (Ehrle, 2001). Custodial grandparents report also losing friendships after bringing their grandchild to social situations (Ehrle, 2001; Giarruso, Feng, Silverstein, & Marenco, 2000). Custodial grandparents also encounter difficulty with the failure of institutional or formal support (e.g., community services, legal protection). In this respect, Ehrle (2001, p. 232) recounts an incident of bias expressed by a family court judge who,

> in an address to an assembly of guardian grandparents, said that grandparents were the very last choice for custody in his court because they were too old to be raising children and they had obviously done a poor job with their own children as evidenced by [the adult child's] irresponsible behavior.

Though such comments may be the exception, they nevertheless suggest that such bias can indeed occur, contributing to the social isolation that some grandparents may feel.

THE IMPACT OF CUSTODIAL GRANDPARENTING ON RELATIONSHIPS WITH OTHERS

Taking on the parenting role strains grandparents' marital relationships (Ehrle & Day, 1994; Shore & Hayslip, 1994). Primary grandparents experience less stress, however, as their spouses' involvement in parenting increases (Musil, 1998). Importantly, the relationship that is most negatively affected by a grandparent becoming a guardian is the grandparent's relationship with the grandchild's parent. In one study, nearly two-thirds of custodial grandparents expressed disappointment in their children, 28% resented them, and over 30% felt taken advantage of by them (Shore & Hayslip, 1994). Not surprisingly, grandparents who have a healthier relationship with their grandchild's parent(s) report feeling less burdened (Pruchno & McKenney, 2000). Other adult children may also feel jealous that their own children are not receiving as much material or emotional support from the grandparent as is the custodial grandchild (Ehrle, 2001). Significantly, most grandparents prefer a fun-loving role with their grandchild, where they can engage their grandchildren without the burden of parental responsibility. By moving into an authority role, custodial grandparents forego the traditional grandparent-grandchild relationship (Emick & Hayslip, 1999). In addition to the role confusion generated, custodial grandparents must grieve the loss of the type of grandparent they envisioned being (Shore & Hayslip, 1994), and in this context, it is not surprising to observe that the quality of the grandparent-grandchild relationship also plays a role in a grandparent's overall adjustment and health (Giarrusso, Silverstein, & Feng, 2000). Additionally, custodial grandparents report being unable to see their noncustodial grandchildren as often as they would like and feel guilty about that inequity (Shore & Hayslip, 1994). Ehrle (2001) also reports that becoming the guardian of one grandchild (or set of grandchildren) can result in family conflicts and, ultimately, alienation from noncustodial grandchildren and their parents.

For custodial grandparents, however, there are numerous challenges to maintaining a supportive network of friends and social contacts. They often sacrifice spending less time with friends because of parenting responsibilities, financial and time constraints, fear of being criticized for their adult child's behavior, and embarrassment about their family situation (Jendrek, 1994). Ehrle (2001) speculates that custodial grandparents feel out of place at events for traditional-aged parents such as PTA meetings. Moreover, given cohort differences in the experience of parenting, they may not have much in common with the parents of their grandchild's friends (Ehrle, 2001).

PARENTING AMONG GRANDPARENTS RAISING GRANDCHILDREN

A number of factors discussed above have been identified as potential sources of increased psychological distress in grandparent caregivers, potentially interfering with their willingness and ability to parent (see Kelley & Whitley, 2003). Other contributing factors in this respect include conflict with the children's parents (see Wohl et al., 2003), the behavior problems of grandchildren, and issues related to both public policies, financial and legal issues (Caliandro & Hughes, 1998; Emick & Hayslip, 1999; Kelley & Damato, 1995; Minkler & Roe, 1993; Yorker, Kelley, Whitley, Lewis, Magis, Bergeron, & Napier, 1998). Although parenting skills training appears to be one of the more widely recommended educational interventions, Pinson-Millburn and colleagues (1996) warn that this training may be met with resistance by grandparents because it implies they may not have adequately parented their adult children. Wohl et al. (2003) feel that prefacing this training with a caveat that stresses how times have changed may help decrease grandparents' defensiveness about this issue, and may help them understand how any caregiver would benefit by gaining greater awareness and skills.

Indeed, given the context of disruptive family events that precede grandparents assuming the care of their grandchildren, the negative impact on parenting skills among such middle-aged and older persons is hardly surprising. With regard to parenting, though grandparents are anticipatorily socialized into their roles (Somary & Stricker, 1998), there is often no such preparation regarding the (re)development of parenting skills that may have been latent for some years. This is especially significant in that for many grandparents, a norm of noninterference (except in crisis situations) with regard to the raising of their grandchildren has been established prior to the resumption of the parental role (Thomas, 1990).

Given the sudden and often stressful circumstances that characterize custodial grandparenting, it is rare to find grandparents whose parental skills are well developed and anchored in current information about (1) parenting practices (e.g., communication, discipline, modeling respect, conflict resolution, problem solving), (2) normal developmental changes in their grandchildren's physical, cognitive, psychosocial, and emotional development, and (3) abnormal childhood disorders such as depression, ADHD, drug use, aggression/acting out behavior, grief at the loss of a parent, self destructive behaviors, or alcoholism. Complicating matters are middle-aged and older grandparents' relative unfamiliarity with issues such as sexually transmitted diseases, drug use, school violence, or peer influences on both children and adolescents, as well as their comparative lack of knowledge about and predisposition not to seek mental health care for either themselves or their grandchildren (Hayslip & Shore, 2000; Silverthorn & Durant, 2000). Significantly, the events that bring about the necessity for care for a grandchild can occur suddenly (e.g., incarceration of the parent; removal of the children due to abuse or neglect), or after a long and difficult period (e.g., death of the parent from AIDS, mental illness, addiction), leaving grandparent caregivers unprepared for such "instant parenting," versus the normal nine-month waiting period most parents experience. This makes further demands on their existing parental skills as they are faced with the additional demands brought about by the difficulties that either they (e.g., depression, poor health) or their grandchildren are experiencing. Complicating matters, grandparents often express shame, guilt, and anxiety due to their adult child's drug addiction, incarceration, or death due to AIDS (Joslin, 2000). Not surprisingly, anger, resentment, or perceived failure as a parent are common in such circumstances.

As Kelley and Whitley (2003) point out, the above discussed physical and mental health issues raise concerns about the quality of the family environment when such grandparents attempt to raise young, active children. As grandparents report concerns about their ability to care for their grandchildren as the former age and/or develop chronic illness and disability (Shore & Hayslip, 1994), both the short-term and long-term impact of custodial grandparenting on such persons' ability to competently raise their grandchildren is of concern, despite the many positive benefits of raising their grandchildren espoused by such grandparents (see above). While some grandparents may require and/or seek minimal updating of their parenting skills, others whose child rearing experiences with their own adult children are either more removed in time or more problematic, or who are raising children with physical or mental health difficulties may need more information, support, and assistance. For such persons, parental skills training that also incorporates support and information about adjustment to one's newly acquired parental role responsibilities, self care/time management skills, as well as information about legal, financial, and health-related services (and their accessibility) is likely to be most beneficial. This is because the above parental role-adjustment and personal issues do not occur in isolation (see Kelley et al., 2001; Smith, 2003; Wohl et al., 2003).

INTERVENTIONS WITH CUSTODIAL GRANDPARENTS

Many researchers and practitioners have noted the need for interventions with custodial grandparents and have recommended implementing support, educational groups, or both, to assist custodial grandparents in coping with, transitioning into, and maintaining these new roles (Chenoweth, 2000; Cox, 2000a; McCallion, Janicki, Grant-Griffin, & Kolomer, 2000; Pinson-Millburn et al., 1996; Strom & Strom, 2000) with positive results being reported for many field studies and support groups. Among other benefits, support groups provide the opportunity for catharsis, whereas education groups can offer information and training related to raising a child in today's society that is uniquely tailored to this population.

In light of the ethical concerns inherent in preventing grandparents from accessing available community-based programs designed explicitly for them (see above), it is not surprising that there has been little experimental intervention work to document the effects of both formal and informal community-based programs on grandparent caregivers and their grandchildren (Hayslip & Patrick, 2003), wherein such work might utilize random assignment to treatment or control groups. By necessity, such work must be based on small samples of convenience, which may not be generalizable to the underlying population of grandparent caregivers. Ideally, it would incorporate both short-term and long-term follow-up efforts to document its efficacy. Such work is best understood in terms of the construct of levels of intervention (Danish, 1981), wherein efforts to effect the adjustment and well being of custodial grandparents could be targeted to the culture at large, the community, and to the interpersonal system which incorporates the grandparent, his/her spouse, as well as the grandchildren that are and are not being cared for by the grandparent. Of course, the impact of such interventions might vary with individual differences in both grandparent and grandchild characteristics such as health status, age, gender, race, and ethnicity. In this context, it is significant that many states are enacting responsive and supportive public policies for these families (Beltran, 2000; Butts, 2000). Yet, challenges remain to educate more states about the need for such policies, as well as to inform policy makers of the informal caregivers in their jurisdiction and the particular obstacles they face.

Many custodial grandparent support groups exist in the United States, but the benefits of these appear to be poorly documented (Strom & Strom, 2000). Anecdotal evidence suggests that custodial grandparents who have the opportunity to meet and interact with other custodial grandparents derive some comfort from doing so, likely mitigating some of the distress associated with their role. It is probable that this especially benefits custodial grandparents who raise children with emotional, behavioral, and learning difficulties as these grandparents often receive less social support than those caring for normal grandchildren (Emick & Hayslip, 1999).

Strom and Strom (2000) note that support groups often fail because they tend to allow members to vent endless frustrations and complaints without moving on to a more positive and constructive focus. Although they are comforted to know that there are other custodial grandparents, members feel helpless and defeated when caught up in a "negative cognitive loop" (see Wohl et al., 2003). Strom and Strom (2000) believe it is important to introduce balance to these groups by emphasizing messages of hope, and celebrating some smaller successes of fellow members along with the members' needs for catharsis. Much more is likely to be gained through learning from others' strengths, rather than dwelling on angry, bitter emotions, as pointed out by Wohl et al. (2003).

Although many mental health professionals recommend education and training for custodial grandparents, few published sources discuss specific interventions of this nature (see Cox, 2000b), and virtually none to date have provided data related to their efficacy. Nonetheless, the need for supportive grandparenting groups has been noted. Hayslip and colleagues (1998) point out that as appropriate models of child-rearing behavior may not exist for these grandparents, it seems especially important to educate them about contemporary child-rearing issues (see above). Furthermore, as custodial grandparenting is a role for which one is seldom prepared, the duration of one's caregiving or the boundaries with other family members may be very unclear and may require new learning (Chenoweth, 2000).

Both Chenoweth (2000) and Strom and Strom (2000) recommend that aspects of support and education be combined in a concurrent group. In contrast, Cox (2000b) recommends that custodial grandparents attend two separate groups simultaneously. As the caregiving role often leaves these grandparents with little unscheduled time, many (e.g., Wohl et al., 2003) believe that membership in two groups simultaneously places an undue burden on them and may be unnecessary. Wohl and colleagues (2003) suggest that aspects of a support group, if facilitated properly, can be present in an education group, if it is well managed. Although this combination would likely benefit many custodial grandparents, it may be especially helpful for those grandparents raising children who have emotional, behavioral, or learning difficulties.

Information and skills training may help remedy problems and prevent future ones (Hayslip et al., 1998), and the support provided may help mitigate the greater distress experience by these caregivers (Wohl et al., 2003). They feel that it is necessary to balance content and education with appropriate emotional support, and feel that when designing custodial grandparent training, areas of content that should be emphasized include (1) parenting skills such as discipline styles, setting limits and consequences, and other contemporary lessons on raising children; (2) communication skills on topics such as how to talk to a teenager, and how to talk to a child's teacher; (3) advocacy issues that include legal/custody questions, and becoming knowledgeable about one's rights; (4) contemporary issues such as drug use and sexuality; and (5) grief and related issues of loss. Because many grandparents are raising children with psychological and behavioral difficulties, sessions focusing on learning disabilities and hyperactivity are also be beneficial (Wohl et al., 2003).

These authors further note that offering support while providing education and skills seems to be more dependent on the skills of the group's leaders/facilitators than on the educational program itself. While allowing grandparents to disclose and share their personal stories, supportive facilitators can establish expectations of growth (Strom & Strom, 2000). It is widely accepted that sharing one's experiences with a group can be a healthy experience when a facilitator encourages constructive self-evaluation.

Furthermore, disclosing personal stories about how they became custodial grandparents, discussing the details of their families, and comparing the memories of raising their adult children with their current experiences can be likened to aspects of the life review process (Butler, 1963; Wohl et al., 2003). Because custodial grandparents often encounter feelings of guilt and regret as they reflect on their role as the parent of their adult children, the life review may provide some perspective in this respect.

A recently published empirical study (Hayslip, 2003) explored the impact of a treatment program whose dual emphasis was on parental skills training and psychosocial adjustment on custodial grandparent parental efficacy, grandchild relationship quality, and personal well-being. It differed from field-based interventions (multi modal home based intervention, see Kelley, Yorker, Whitley, Sipe, & Yorker, 2001), which understandably lack random assignment to groups as an attribute. The Hayslip study (2003) found that for training participants (relative to controls), Negative Affect scores (irritation/difficulty with the grandchild's negative behaviors) decreased over time (pre-versus post-program), Parental Self Efficacy increased over time, as did the rated Quality of the Relationship with one's Grandchild, while Parental Role Strain increased over time, as did both Financial Strain and Depression. Though the magnitude of these effects was modest, they do document the extent to which the parental skills and psychosocial adjustment of grandparents can be effected by purposefully designed interventions targeting for many grandparents what have been heretofore unspoken issues regarding the demands of raising a grandchild. For many grandparents, it may be that the evocation of the skills that they acquired over the course of the program made matters at home somewhat more tense, as might be the case when issues regarding the impact of their parenting roles on their marriages, relationships with friends, frustrations with service providers, social service agencies, school personnel, or with the adult child are aired for the first time, or when they became aware of the difficulty in changing their grandchild's behavior. It may also be that grandparents were in some cases reactivating previous parenting styles that were perhaps somewhat traditional and/or authority-oriented, making their interactions in some cases with their grandchildren more difficult. This may explain the small, yet reliable increases in parental role strain, financial strain, and depression over time in training participants relative to waiting list controls. Thus, the program may have brought to the surface previously ineffective ways of interacting with their adult children when the latter were young, heightened grandparents' awareness of the child-rearing task before them, or allowed them the freedom to discuss their negative feelings and frustrations at having to parent again. Therapeutically, this can be advantageous in that many grandparents are able to test the validity of many of the assumptions they had previously held about parenting, and are able to see their advantages and disadvantages in the context of their daily interactions with their grandchildren and weekly interactions with one another. Comparatively speaking, there was some indication (see Hayslip, 2003) that regarding parental efficacy, quality and satisfaction with grandchild relationships, life satisfaction, and Negative Affect, persons who lacked the presumed benefits of parental skills/psychosocial adjustment training actually *worsened* over time. It could be argued that in some respects, this program made grandparents more attentive to the difficulties of raising a grandchild, but was less effective in providing easily implemented solutions to such problems, especially when the sources of such difficulties were beyond the ability and resources of many grandparents to control, e.g., difficulties with the school system, legal uncertainties over custody, unresponsive child protective services, grief over a "broken" family system. Significantly, in this respect, grandparents felt no greater sense of empowerment after training. Indeed, as with support groups (see Smith, 2003), it could be argued that parental and psychosocial skills training can be counterproductive for some persons, and in this respect parallels in part the findings discussed by Roberto and Qualls (2003) regarding caregiver respite programs. Yet, there is much benefit in the discomfort one feels when existing beliefs are challenged and heretofore unspoken feelings are aired (Hayslip, 2003). While training can allow some grandparents to become more open to change, such openness is not without its costs (see Wohl et al., 2003).

Indeed, interventions with custodial grandparents should be thought of in terms of alternatives to a single best approach that works for everyone, i.e., individual and group therapy, respite programs, support groups (see Cohen & Pyle, 2000), community education. Indeed, based on empirical data gathered from grandparent caregivers, the content, leadership (peer vs. professional), involvement by grandchildren, nature of group goals, should all be purposefully heterogeneous (Smith, 2003).

FUTURE DIRECTIONS IN CUSTODIAL GRANDPARENTING

Longitudinal research, especially of a prospective nature, may yield important understandings regarding the antecedents of parental styles and coping mechanisms employed by custodial grandparents, as the dynamics of such relationships are likely to be in flux. To date, only a handful of such studies exist (Hayslip, Emick, & Henderson, 2003; Minkler et al., 1997; Strawbridge, Wallhagen, Shema, & Kaplan, 1997). Such data may provide important insights for the targets of psychosocial interventions with custodial grandparents.

Interventions that target both grandparent caregivers and grandchildren may be the most effective. In this respect, it is noteworthy to observe that a developmental sense, we know little about the consequences in adulthood of having been raised by one's grandparents. Such persons may hold more positive attitudes toward aging or may be more effective parents. Moreover, the long-term impact of having raised a grandchild later in life on such grandparents is unknown at present. As grandparents raising grandchildren exhibiting problems report the most distress (Hayslip et al., 1998), further work regarding factors contributing to the problems displayed by such grandchildren may prove useful in the development of appropriate services for problem grandchildren and their grandparents. Moreover, we know little about cultural variations in custodial grandparenting (see Toledo et al., 2000), and as noted above, virtually all such studies involve primarily grandmothers and few grandfathers. Information speaking to these issues, to those relating to family system-related processes in grandparent-headed families, and to the diversity among custodial grandparents, will be valuable in the design and implementation of helping efforts directed to grandparents and the grandchildren they are raising. Over the last two decades, we have made much progress in our knowledge of and sensitivity to grandparents who raise their grandchildren, but there is much that we do not yet know.

REFERENCES

Ainsworth, M. (1989). Attachments beyond infancy. *American Psychologist, 44,* 709-716.

Antonucci, T. (1990). Social supports and social relationships. In R. Binstock & L. George (Eds.), *The handbook of aging and the social sciences (3rd ed.)* (pp. 205-226). San Diego, CA: Academic Press.

Baltes, P. B. (1997). On the incomplete architecture of human ontogeny: Selection, optimization, and compensation as foundation of developmental theory. *American Psychologist, 52,* 366-380.

Baird, A. (2003). Through my eyes: Service needs of grandparents who raise their grandchildren from the perspective of a custodial grandmother. In B. Hayslip & J. Patrick (Eds.), *Working with custodial grandparents* (pp. 59-68). New York: Springer.

Beltran, A. (2000). Grandparents and other relatives raising children: Supportive public policies. *The Public Policy and Aging Report, Summer, 2000,* pp. 1, 3-7.

Bryson (2001, November). *New Census Bureau data on grandparents raising grandchildren.* Paper presented at the Annual Scientific Meeting of the Gerontological Society of America. Chicago, IL.

Burnette, D. (1999a). Physical and emotional well-being of custodial grandparents in Latino families. *American Journal of Orthopsychiatry, 69*, 305-317.

Burnette, D. (1999b). Social relationships of Latino grandparent caregivers: A role theory perspective. *The Gerontologist, 39*, 49-58.

Burnette, D. (2000). Latino grandparents rearing children with special needs: Effects of depressive symptomology. *Journal of Gerontological Social Work, 33*, 1-16.

Burton, L. M. (1992). Black grandparents rearing children of drug-addicted parents: Stressors, outcomes, and social service needs. *The Gerontologist, 32*, 744-751.

Burton, L., & DeVries, C. (1993). Challenges and rewards: African American grandparents as surrogate parents. *Generations, 17*, 51-54.

Butler, R. (1963). The life review: An interpretation of reminiscence in the aged. *Psychiatry, 26*, 65-76.

Butts, D. (2000). Organizational advocacy as a factor in public policy regarding custodial grandparenting. In B. Hayslip & R. Goldberg-Glen (Eds.), *Grandparents raising grandchildren: Theoretical, empirical and clinical issues* (pp. 341-350). New York: Springer.

Caliandro, G., & Hughes, C. (1998). The experience of being a grandmother who is the primary caregiver for her HIV-positive grandchild. *Nursing Research, 47*, 107-113.

Carstensen, L. L. (1995). Evidence for a life-span theory of socioemotional selectivity. *Current Directions in Psychological Science, 4*, 151-156.

Casper, L., & Bryson, K. (1998). *Co-resident grandparents and their grandchildren: Grandparent maintained families.* U.S. Census Bureau: Washington, DC. U.S. Government Printing Office.

Chenoweth, L. (2000). Grandparent education. In B. Hayslip & R. Goldberg-Glen (Eds.), *Grandparents raising grandchildren: Theoretical, empirical and clinical issues* (pp. 307-326). New York: Springer.

Cohen, C. S., & Pyle, R. (2000). Support groups in the lives of grandmothers. In C. Cox (Ed.), *To grandmother's house we go and stay: Perspectives on custodial grandparents* (pp. 235-252). New York: Springer.

Cox, C. (2000a). Why grandchildren are going and staying at grandmother's house and what happens when they get there. In C. Cox (Ed.), *To grandmother's house we go and stay: Perspectives on custodial grandparents* (pp. 3-19). New York: Springer.

Cox, C. (2000b). Empowering grandparents raising grandchildren. In C. Cox (Ed.), *To grandmother's house we go and stay: Perspectives on custodial grandparents* (pp. 253-268). New York: Springer.

Cox, C., Brooks, L. R., & Valcarcel, C. (2000). Culture and caregiving: A study of Latino grandparents. In C. Cox (Ed.), *To grandmother's house we go and stay: Perspectives on custodial grandparents* (pp. 215-233). New York: Springer.

Crowther, M., & Rodriguez, R. (2003). A stress and coping model of custodial grandparenting among African Americans. In B. Hayslip & J. Patrick (Eds.), *Working with custodial grandparents* (pp. 145-162). New York: Springer.

Danish, S. (1981). Life span development and intervention: A necessary link. *Counseling Psychologist, 9*, 40-43.

Emick, M., & Hayslip, B. (1996). Custodial grandparenting: New roles for middle aged and older adults. *International Journal of Aging and Human Development, 43*, 135-154.

Emick, M., & Hayslip, B. (1999). Custodial grandparenting: Stresses, coping skills, and relationships with grandchildren. *International Journal of Aging and Human Development, 48,* 35-62.

Ehrle, G. M. (2001). Grandchildren as moderator variables in the family: Social, physiological, and intellectual development of grandparents who are raising them. *Family Development and Intellectual Functions, 12,* 223-241.

Ehrle, G. M., & Day, H. D. (1994). Adjustment and family functioning of grandmothers raising their grandchildren. *Contemporary Family Therapy, 16,* 67-82.

Fuller-Thomson, E., & Minkler, M. (2000). The mental and physical health of grandmothers who are raising their grandchildren. *Journal of Mental Health and Aging, 6,* 311-323.

Fuller-Thomson, E., & Minkler, M. (2001). American grandparents providing extensive child care to their grandchildren: Prevalence and profile. *The Gerontologist, 41,* 201-209.

Gatti, F. L., & Musatti, T. (1999). Grandmothers' involvement in grandchildren's care: Attitudes, feelings, and emotions. *Family Relations, 48,* 35-42.

Giarrusso, R., Silverstein, M., & Feng, D. (2000). Psychological costs and benefits of raising grandchildren: Evidence from a national survey of grandparents. In C. Cox (Ed.), *To grandmother's house we go and stay: Perspectives on custodial grandparents* (pp. 71-90). New York: Springer.

Giarrusso, R., Feng, D., Silverstein, M., & Marenco, A. (2000). Primary and secondary stressors of raising grandchildren: Evidence from a national survey. *Journal of Mental Health and Aging, 6,* 291-310.

Goodman, C., & Silverstein, M. (2002). Grandparents raising grandchildren: Family structure and well being in culturally diverse families. *The Gerontologist, 42,* 676-689.

Hagestad, G. (1988). Demographic change and the life course: Some emerging trends in the family realm. *Family Relations, 37,* 405-410.

Harper, W., & Hardesty, P. (2001). Differentiating characteristics and needs of minority grandparent caregivers. *Journal of Ethnic and Cultural Diversity in Social Work, 9,* 133-150.

Hayslip, B. (2003). The impact of a psychosocial intervention on parental efficacy, grandchild relationship quality, and well being among grandparents raising grandchildren. In B. Hayslip & J. Patrick (Eds.), *Working with custodial grandparents* (pp. 163-178). New York: Springer.

Hayslip, B., Emick, M., & Henderson, C. (2002). Temporal variations in the experience of custodial grandparenting: A short term longitudinal approach. *Journal of Applied Gerontology, 21,* 139-156.

Hayslip, B., Henderson, C., & Shore, R. J. (2003). The structure of grandparental role meaning. *Journal of Adult Development, 10,* 1-11.

Hayslip, B., & Patrick, J. (2003). Custodial grandparenting viewed from within a life-span perspective. In B. Hayslip & J. Patrick (Eds.), *Working with custodial grandparents* (pp. 3-12). New York: Springer.

Hayslip, B., & Shore, R. J. (2000). Custodial grandparenting and mental health services. *Journal of Mental Health and Aging, 6,* 367-384.

Hayslip, B., Shore, R. J., Henderson, C., & Lambert, P. (1998). Custodial grandparenting and grandchildren with problems: Their impact on role satisfaction and role meaning. *Journal of Gerontology: Social Sciences, 53B*, S164-S174.

Hirshorn, B., Van Meter, J., & Brown, D. (2000). When grandparents raise their grandchildren due to substance abuse: Responding to a uniquely destabilizing factor. In B. Hayslip & R. Goldberg-Glen (Eds.), *Grandparents raising grandchildren: Theoretical, empirical and clinical perspectives* (pp. 269-288). New York: Springer.

Jendrek, M. (1994). Grandparents who parent their grandchildren: Circumstances and decisions. *The Gerontologist, 34*, 206-216.

Joslin, D. (2000). Emotional well-being among grandparents affected and orphaned by HIV disease. In B. Hayslip & R. Goldberg-Glen (Eds.), *Grandparents raising grandchildren: Theoretical, empirical and clinical perspectives* (pp. 87-106). New York: Springer.

Joslin, D. (2002). *Invisible caregivers: Older adults raising children in the wake of HIV/AIDS*. Columbia, NY: Columbia University Press.

Kahn, R., & Antonucci, T. (1980). Convoys over the life course: Attachment, roles, and social support. In P.B. Baltes & O.G. Brim (Eds.), *Life-span development and behavior: Volume 3* (pp. 254-286). New York: Academic Press.

Kelley, S. J., & Damato, E. G. (1995). Grandparents as primary caregivers. *Maternal Child Nursing, 20*, 326-332.

Kelley, S. J., & Whitley, D. (2003). Psychological distress and physical health problems in grandparents raising grandchildren: Development of an empirically based intervention model. In B. Hayslip & J. Patrick (Eds.), *Working with custodial grandparents* (pp. 127-144). New York: Springer.

Kelley, S. J., Whitley, D. M., Sipe, T. A., & Yorker, B. C. (2000). Psychological distress in grandmother kinship care providers: The role of resources, social support and physical health. *Child Abuse & Neglect, 24*, 311-321.

Kelley, S. J., Whitley, D. M., Sipe, T. A., & Yorker, B. C. (October, 2001). *Results of an interdisciplinary intervention to improve the well-being and functioning of grandparents raising grandchildren*. Paper presented at the American Public Health Association Annual Meeting, Atlanta, GA.

Kirby, J., & Kaneda, T. (2002). Health insurance and family structure: The case of adolescents in skipped generation families. *Medical Care Research and Review, 59*, 146-165.

Kolomer, S., McCallion, P., & Overeynder, J. (2003). Why support groups help: Successful interventions for grandparent caregivers of children with developmental disabilities. In B. Hayslip & J. Patrick (Eds.), *Working with custodial grandparents* (pp. 111-126). New York: Springer.

McCallion, P., Janicki, M., Grant-Griffin, L., & Kolomer, S. (2000). Grandparent caregivers II: Service needs and service provision issues. *Journal of Gerontological Social Work, 33*, 57-84.

McKinney, J., McGrew, K., & Nelson, I. (2003). Grandparent caregivers to children with developmental disabilities: Added challenges. In B. Hayslip & J. Patrick (Eds.), *Working with custodial grandparents* (pp. 93-110). New York: Springer.

Minkler, M., & Fuller-Thomson, E. (2001). Physical and mental health status of American grandparents providing extensive child care to their grandchildren. *Journal of the American Medical Women's Association, 56*, 199-205.

Minkler, M., Fuller-Thomson, E., Miller, D., & Driver, D. (1997). Depression in grandparents raising grandchildren: Results of a national longitudinal study. *Archives of Family Medicine, 6,* 445-452.

Minkler, M., & Roe, K. M. (1993). *Grandmothers as caregivers: Raising children of the crack cocaine epidemic.* Newbury Park, CA: Sage.

Minkler, M., Roe, K. M., & Robertson-Beckley, R. J. (1994). Raising grandchildren from crack-cocaine households: Effects on family & friendship ties of African-American women. *American Journal of Orthopsychiatry, 64,* 20-29.

Musil, C. (1998). Health, stress, coping, and social support in grandmother caregivers. *Health Care for Women International, 19,* 101-114.

Nelson, E., & Dannefer, D. (1992). Aged heterogeneity: Fact or fiction. The fate of diversity in gerontological research. *The Gerontologist, 32,* 17-23.

Patrick, J., & Hayslip, B. (2003). Epilogue: The next stage in helping custodial grandparents. In B. Hayslip & J. Patrick (Eds.), *Working with custodial grandparents* (pp. 277-282). New York: Springer.

Pearlin, L., Mullan, J., Semple, S., & Skaff, M. (1990). Caregiving and the stress process: An overview of concepts and their measures. *The Gerontologist, 20,* 583-592.

Pinson-Millburn, M., Fabian, E., Schlossberg, N., & Pyle, M. (1996). Grandparents raising grandchildren. *Journal of Counseling and Development, 74,* 548-554.

Pruchno, R. (1999). Raising grandchildren: The experiences of Black and White grandmothers. *The Gerontologist, 39,* 209-221.

Pruchno, R., & McKinney, D. (2000). Living with grandchildren: The effects of custodial and co-resident households on the mental health of grandmothers. *Journal of Mental Health and Aging, 6,* 269-289.

Roberto, K., & Qualls, S. (2003). Intervention strategies for grandparents raising grandchildren: lessons learned from the caregiving literature. In B. Hayslip & J. Patrick (Eds.), *Working with custodial grandparents* (pp. 13-26). New York: Springer.

Robinson, M. M., Kropf, N. P., & Myers, L. L. (2000). Grandparents raising grandchildren in rural communities. *Journal of Mental Health and Aging, 6,* 353-365.

Shore, R. J., & Hayslip, B. (1994). Custodial grandparenting: Implications for children's development. In A. Gottfried & A. Gottfried (Eds.), *Redefining families: Implications for children's development* (pp. 171-218). New York: Plenum.

Silverstein, N., & Vehvilainen, L. (2000). Grandparents and schools: Issues and potential challenges. In C. Cox (Ed.), *To grandmother's house we go and stay: Perspectives on custodial grandparents* (pp. 268-283). New York: Springer.

Silverthorn, P., & Durant, S. (2000). Custodial grandparenting and the difficult child: Learning from the parenting literature (pp. 47-64). In B. Hayslip & R. Goldberg-Glen (Eds.), *Grandparents raising grandchildren: Theoretical, empirical and clinical perspectives* (pp. 47-64). New York: Springer.

Smith, G. (2003). How grandparents view support groups: An exploratory study. In B. Hayslip & J. Patrick (Eds.), *Working with custodial grandparents* (pp. 69-92). New York: Springer.

Solomon, J. C., & Marx, J. (1995). "To grandmother's house we go": Health and school adjustment of children raised solely by grandparents. *The Gerontologist, 35,* 386-394.

Somary, K., & Stricker, G. (1998). Becoming a grandparent: A longitudinal study of expectations and early experiences as a function of sex and lineage. *The Gerontologist, 38,* 53-61.

Strawbridge, W. J., Wallhagen, M. I., Shema, S. J., & Kaplan, G. A. (1997). New burdens or more of the same? Comparing grandparent, spouse, and adult-child caregivers. *The Gerontologist, 37,* 505-510.

Stroebe, M., & Schut, H. (1999). The dual process model of coping with bereavement: Rationale and description. *Death Studies, 23,* 197-224.

Strom, R., & Strom, S. (2000). Goals for grandparent caregivers and support groups. In B. Hayslip & R. Goldberg-Glen (Eds.), *Grandparents raising grandchildren: Theoretical, empirical and clinical perspectives* (pp. 171-218). New York: Springer.

Thoits, P. A. (1995). Stress, coping, and social support processes: Where are we? What next? *Journal of Health and Social Behavior, Special Review, 12,* 53-79.

Thomas, J. L. (1990). The grandparent role: A double bind. *International Journal of Aging and Human Development, 31,* 169-177.

Toledo, R., Hayslip, B., Emick, M., Toledo, C., & Henderson, C. (2000). Cross-cultural differences in custodial grandparenting. In B. Hayslip & R. Goldberg-Glen (Eds.), *Grandparents raising grandchildren: Theoretical, empirical and clinical perspectives* (pp. 107-124). New York: Springer.

Uhlenberg, P., & Kirby, J. (1998). Grandparenthood over time: Historical and demographic trends. In M. Szionovacz (Ed.), *Handbook on grandparenthood* (pp. 23-39). Westport, CN: Greenwood Press.

Unger, J. B., McAvay, G., Bruce, M. L., Berman, L., & Seeman, T. (1999). Variation in the impact of social network characteristics on physical functioning in elderly persons: McArthur studies of successful aging. *Journal of Gerontology: Social Sciences, 54B,* S245-251.

U.S. Bureau of the Census (2003). *Grandparents living with grandchildren: Census 2000 Brief* (pp. 1-10). Washington, DC: U.S. Government Printing Office. www.census.gov.

Wohl, E., Lahner, J., & Jooste, J. (2003). Group processes among grandparents raising grandchildren. In B. Hayslip & J. Patrick (Eds.), *Working with custodial grandparents* (pp. 195-212). New York: Springer.

Yorker, B. C., Kelley, S. J., Whitley, D. M., Lewis, A., Magis, J., Bergeron, A., & Napier, C. (1998). Custodial relationships of grandparents raising grandchildren: Results of a home-based intervention study. *Juvenile and Family Court Journal, 49,* 15-25.

Caregiver Stress Among Grandparents Raising Grandchildren: The Functional Role of Social Support

Laura Landry-Meyer
Jean M. Gerard
Jacqueline R. Guzell

SUMMARY. Drawing from family stress theory, this study examined the associations among caregiver stress, social support, and stress outcomes measured by life satisfaction and generativity among grandparents raising grandchildren. Social support was hypothesized to moderate the association between caregiver stress and stress outcome indicators. Using survey data from a non-probability sample of 133 grandparent caregivers with full-time responsibility of raising at least one grand-

Laura Landry-Meyer is Assistant Professor, Human Development and Family Studies, Bowling Green State University. Jean M. Gerard is Assistant Professor, Human Development and Family Studies, Bowling Green State University, 206 Johnston Hall, Bowling Green, OH 43403-0254. Jacqueline R. Guzell is Assistant Professor, Human Development and Family Studies, Bowling Green State University, 206 Johnston Hall, Bowling Green, OH 43403-0254.

Address correspondence to: Laura Landry-Meyer, Human Development and Family Studies, Bowling Green State University, Bowling Green, OH 43403-0254 (E-mail: landrym@bgnet.bgsu.edu).

This research was supported by a grant from College of Education and Human Development Interdisciplinary Research Fund at Bowling Green State University.

[Haworth co-indexing entry note]: "Caregiver Stress Among Grandparents Raising Grandchildren: The Functional Role of Social Support." Landry-Meyer, Laura, Jean M. Gerard, and Jacqueline R. Guzell. Co-published simultaneously in *Marriage & Family Review* (The Haworth Press, Inc.) Vol. 37, No. 1/2, 2005, pp. 171-190; and: *Challenges of Aging on U.S. Families: Policy and Practice Implications* (ed: Richard K. Caputo) The Haworth Press, Inc., 2005, pp. 171-190. Single or multiple copies of this article are available for a fee from The Haworth Document Delivery Service [1-800-HAWORTH, 9:00 a.m. - 5:00 p.m. (EST). E-mail address: docdelivery@haworthpress.com].

171

child, regression analysis demonstrated that caregiver stress is associated negatively with life satisfaction and generativity. Informal and formal social support was found to have a beneficial influence on stress outcomes that generalizes to grandparent caregiver participants regardless of the amount of stress they experience. Contrary to predictions, social support did not buffer the association between caregiver stress and life satisfaction nor the association between caregiver stress and generativity. A high degree of perceived informal support was found to function as a detriment to grandparents under conditions of high stress through lowered generativity. Results suggest the need to examine the functional role of social support in the caregiving context. *[Article copies available for a fee from The Haworth Document Delivery Service: 1-800-HAWORTH. E-mail address: <docdelivery@haworthpress.com> Website: <http://www.HaworthPress.com> © 2005 by The Haworth Press, Inc. All rights reserved.]*

KEYWORDS. Grandparent caregivers, social support, stress, life satisfaction, generativity

INTRODUCTION

The number of grandparents raising grandchildren has steadily increased over the past few decades. Saluter (1992) reported a 44% increase in the number of children residing with grandparents or other relatives between 1980 and 1990. More recent data suggests that approximately 5.6 million grandparents maintain households that include children younger than age 18 (Roberto & Qualls, 2003). Using national survey data, Fuller-Thomson and Minkler (2000) estimate that 14.5% of grandmothers have raised a grandchild for six months or more.

The increase in grandparent caregivers is cause for concern, given the stress associated with parenting at an unexpected life stage. The family role transition from grandparent to surrogate parent inherently involves life-stage stressors such as financial issues (e.g., parenting and retirement are incongruent), role ambiguity (e.g., being a grandparent to some grandchildren while being a parent to other grandchildren), and personal adjustments to daily lifestyle. Grandparent caregiving is linked to several negative outcomes including decreased peer-network interaction and social isolation, depression, and lowered life satisfaction (Burton, 1992; Caputo, 2000; Fuller-Thomson & Minkler, 2000; Jendrek,

1993; Kelley, Whitley, Sipe, & Yorker, 2000). Most of the research has studied the effect of stress on grandparent caregivers and has neglected social support resources that may moderate stress outcomes. In light of the stress associated with the resumption of the parenting role, it is important to identify social support resources that may facilitate positive development among grandparent caregivers.

Social support is an important component in determining the way in which a grandparent interprets the stress of raising a grandchild (Kelley et al., 2000). Theoretically, social support is a resource that buffers the relationship between caregiver stress and well-being (Crowther & Rodriguez, 2003; Miller, Townsend, Carpenter, Montgomery, Stull, & Young, 2001). However, few investigators have actually tested this proposition using formal statistical techniques and, to date, there is limited evidence supporting this proposition for grandparent caregivers (Chappell & Reid, 2002; Crowther & Rodriguez, 2003). Using family stress theory, this investigation tests whether social support buffers the association between caregiver stress and outcomes of well-being as measured by life satisfaction and generativity. A primary focus is on both informal and formal social support to determine the role of support mechanisms in alleviating stress associated with grandparent caregiving.

OVERVIEW

Recent grandparent caregiving studies have used stress theory as a guiding framework (Crowther & Rodriguez, 2003; Giarusso, Feng, Silverstein, & Marenco, 2000; Sands & Goldberg-Glen, 2000) and the gerontological caregiving literature has utilized a stress process model to explain the context for families (e.g., Pearlin, Mullan, Semple, & Skaff, 1990). This model and family stress theory demarcates the role of resources, such as social support on the stressor. Social support is seen to moderate the effect of caregiver stress. As a stress coping resource in the caregiving context, the type of social support viewed as most effective is in dispute (Miller et al., 2001). Recent caregiving investigations have found mixed and unexpected relationships among stressors and social support (Crowther & Rodriguez, 2003; Miller et al., 2001) leading to the question: does social support help to alleviate the stress of raising a grandchild?

Family stress theory is used to guide this investigation with a focus on the role of social support as a coping resource. The emphasis on the familial environment is rooted in family stress theory, a variant of broader stress theory that focuses specifically on crises that incapacitate a family system (Hill, 1949). From this perspective, a stressor includes a non-normative transition in the family life cycle. The re-parenting role that the grandparent assumes is a non-normative transition. Re-parenting stress is viewed through caregiving obligations that increase daily demands, restrict freedom and flexibility, create financial burden or worry, and elicit ongoing concerns about grandchildren's well-being (Landry-Meyer & Newman, in press). These obligations are considered stressors that trigger the need for coping and impact life satisfaction and adult personality development.

Social Support

Social support is considered a resource that a grandparent caregiver brings to the environment to cope with a stressor (Crowther & Rodriguez, 2003). To explore social support in the context of grandparents raising grandchildren, two types of social support are examined: informal and formal. Both types of social support refer to individuals having or feeling a sense of assistance. Informal support is conceptualized as support received from family, friends, and a confidant or partner. Formal social support is "governed by contractual or paid arrangements rather than affiliation and obligation norms" (Litwak, 1985 as reported by Miller et al., 2001, p. S250). As a multidimensional construct, these categories are further delineated into specific types of support: the social network, perceived support, and enacted support.

The social network. The social network is comprised of "the connections that individuals have to significant others in their social environments" (Barrera, 1986, p. 415). The social network is an important resource to grandparent caregivers as they adapt to their re-parenting role (Minkler, Roe, & Robertson-Beckley, 1994). From a network of community services to a circle of family and friends, the network is viewed as salient in the amount of resources a grandparent may have available when faced with the stress of raising a grandchild. Minkler and colleagues (1994) found that despite a high degree of social embeddedness prior to raising a grandchild, many grandparent caregivers report decreased contact with some support members after assuming caregiving. Specifically, for friend networks, approximately one-half of grandparents ceased having contact with a friend due to responsibilities associated with raising a grandchild.

The social network is similar to Erikson's (1963) conceptualization of radius of significant others. Although social networks are regarded as highly important for grandparents raising grandchildren, there is a potential drawback to having a strong social network. Erikson postulates that an individual's network of relationships determines not only the resources that are available, but also the demands that are placed upon that individual. A social network may be non-supportive. Grandparent caregivers in strong social networks are more likely to be affected by the views and opinions of its members than grandparents without such a dense network, and this may or may not be compatible with the grandparent's re-parenting role.

Perceived support. Perceived support refers to an individual's perception of the availability and adequacy of one's network. Despite support network membership, relatively few grandparent caregivers perceive themselves as receiving consistent and reliable support (Burton, 1992). Many are uncomfortable seeking support from friends who are no longer parenting (Jendrek, 1993). This perception is related to grandparent caregivers feeling off-time when compared to their same-age peers (Landry-Meyer & Newman, in press).

A belief that older adults shun the use of 'charity' makes grandparent caregivers' perception of social services salient. Perception of formal social support incorporates the attitude grandparent caregivers have about the availability and use of social service delivery systems. Often grandparent caregivers do not access social services because they do not know that these types of services exist nor do not want to accept social welfare (Landry-Meyer, 1999a).

Enacted support. Enacted support refers to actual support received, such as type and amount of services or type and amount of supportive interactions such as physical comforting, receiving advice, or receiving financial help (Vaux & Harrison, 1985). Grandparent caregivers have been found to have high social service needs, yet few studies have determined effectiveness of service usage (Landry-Meyer, 1999b). In terms of support received from an informal network, mixed results have emerged. Minkler and colleagues (1994) found that the majority of grandmothers in their study were members of a dense support network and received high levels of enacted support. In contrast, Burton (1992) found that 97% of the grandparent caregivers in her study received little to no familial support despite large support networks. Determining the effect of these types of support mechanisms on re-parenting stress becomes central to strengthening the grandparent-grandchild family structure.

Stress Outcomes

Outcomes reflect the impact of the stressor on an individual's well-being as shaped by the interaction between the stressor and the resource. With a focus on social support as a moderator, stress outcomes are viewed as positive adjustments. For this investigation, life satisfaction and generativity were used as outcome measures. Life satisfaction is widely used as an outcome measure and refers to a general feeling of well-being based on one's evaluation of life.

Generativity was also used as an outcome variable. The concept of life satisfaction gives little attention to the active engagement of life (Fisher, 1995) whereas generativity involves the way in which an individual actualizes their sense of well-being. Generativity, as conceptualized by Erikson, is widely understood to involve caring for future generations. In this sense, caring for a grandchild is a reflection of active engagement with life (Strawbridge, Wallhagen, & Cohen, 2002). Generative tasks usually include nurturing and caregiving, but can also include intellectual and creative activities (McAdams & de St. Aubin, 1992). While these tasks are worthy pursuits, they may be incompatible with non-normative family transitions, such as re-parenting. Grandparents involved in re-parenting may be less likely to have time for some generative pursuits. The inability to participate in such activities may limit their resolution of this psychosocial task.

The transition to full-time parenting is a stressful life event. Drawing from family stress theory, this study examined the associations among caregiver stress, social support, and stress outcomes measured by life satisfaction and generativity among grandparents raising grandchildren. Social support was hypothesized to moderate the association between caregiver stress and indicators of stress outcomes.

METHODS

Participants

Participants were drawn from the Grandparent Family Project, a study of grandparents raising a grandchild in the northwest Ohio and surrounding areas. The sample consisted of 133 grandparents and great-grandparents who met the following criteria: (a) the grandparent had primary caregiving responsibilities for one or more grandchildren, (b) the grandchild resided in the grandparent's household, and (c) the grandchild's biological parent did not reside in the grandparent's household. Participants were recruited through social service agencies; those who met eligibility requirements completed an informed-consent form and survey. Participants received a $20 gift certificate as an incentive.

Among participants, 91% were female, 9% male; 53% were married, 26% divorced, 14% widowed, 4% were single/never married and 3% separated. Close to 19% of participants did not graduate from high school and 33% had annual household incomes of less than $19,000 for an average household size of three individuals. Slightly over half of the grandparents were employed. In terms of ethnicity, 79% of participants were Caucasian and 21% were African-American.

The average number of grandchildren raised by participants was 1.7. Fifty-five percent of grandparents reported raising one grandchild, 29% reported two, 7% reported three, and 10% reported raising four or more children. One-fourth of the grandchildren in these households were under the age of five, 35% were 5 to 9 years old, 30% were 10 to 14 years old, and 10% were 15 to 19 years old. Grandchildren were divided equally across gender. Ethnicity of grandchildren was more varied than participants (63% Caucasian, 25% African American, 10% bi-racial, and 2% other). The average length of time children were in the care of grandparents was 56 months and 94% of participants had a custodial relationship with the grandchild.

Measures

Caregiver stress. Caregiver stress was measured using a modified version of the 18-item Parental Stress Index, an established measure with documented evidence of reliability and validity (Berry & Jones, 1995). Modifications were necessary to adapt individual items so that they reflected the degree of stress associated with re-parenting rather than parenting. For example, the item "Having children leaves little time and flexibility in my life" was modified to "Raising grandchildren leaves little time and flexibility in my life." The five-point response ranged from *strongly disagree* (1) to *strongly agree* (5). Cronbach alpha for the scale was .90 with average score of 2.3 ($SD = 6.2$).

Social support. Social support was measured using the broad categories of informal and formal social support. Within each broach category, specific types of support were measured.

Informal social support. Three dimensions of informal social support were assessed: network, perceived, and enacted. Network was measured asking to quantify the number in their support network as well as using a modified version of the Lubben Social Network Scale (Lubben, 1988). Participants were asked to indicate the number of family, friends, and confidants they had contact with during a specified time period. Two items in the original scale were omitted based on the context of grandparent caregivers. Scores for the eight items were summed so that higher values reflected greater network density. Average participant score was 25.7 (*SD* = 6.1) for the entire scale with family subscale average 10.3 (*SD* = 2.9), friend average 8.3 (*SD* = 3.0), and confidante average 7.1 (*SD* = 6.1). Cronbach alpha for the measure was .75.

Perceived informal social support was measured using the 12-item Multidimensional Scale of Perceived Social Support (Zimet, Dahlmen, Zimet, & Farley, 1988). The MSPSS is designed to measure the degree of perceived social support with three subscales: family, friends, and a confidante. The seven-point response format ranged from *very strongly disagree* (1) to *very strongly agree* (7). Cronbach alpha was .93 with an average scale score of 5.5 (*SD* = 1.1). Average subscales scores were as follows: family = 5.3 (*SD* = 1.5), friend = 5.4 (*SD* = 1.3), confidant = 5.9 (*SD* = 1.3).

Informal enacted social support was assessed by asking participants to identify the number of individuals in their support network who have provided support to the participant during the past year. On average, participants received assistance from 5.5 individuals in the past year (*SD* = 7.5).

Formal social support. Two dimensions of formal social support were assessed: perceived and enacted. Perceived formal support was measured using the Attitudes Toward Use of Formal Help or Community Services (Lai, 1996). This 14-item instrument assesses the degree to which respondents agree with various statements about the use of professional and community services, such as, "Although there are community service organizations for people with needs, you don't think they are useful to you." The five-point response format ranged from *strongly disagree* (1) to *strongly agree* (5). Cronbach alpha for this measure was .74.

Enacted formal support was assessed using a 13-item index created for the study based on a similar measure used in a statewide grandparent caregiver survey (Downey, 1998). The index represents the number of formal services utilized by grandparents and their grandchildren in a checklist format. Sample items are church-related programs, medical services, legal services, and counseling services. Internal consistency of the index was good (α = .73).

Stress outcomes. Stress outcomes were assessed using life satisfaction and generativity. Life satisfaction was measured using the 18-item Life Satisfaction Index-Z (LSIZ) developed by Neugarten, Havighurst, and Tobin (1961). LSIZ has been used extensively with older adults and was chosen for its gerontological focus. Respondents are asked to rate whether they *disagree* (0) or *agree* (1) with each statement or are *unsure* (2) about any of the statements. Cronbach alpha for this measure was .75 with an average score of .81 (*SD* = .26).

Generativity was measured using a modified version of the Loyola Generativity Scale (LGS) to assess individual differences in adults' generative concern with responses ranging from *never* (1) to *very often* (4) (McAdams & de St. Aubin, 1992). Thus, higher scores reflect a greater sense of generativity. Cronbach alpha for the scale was .83 with average score of 2.39 (*SD* = .43).

Control variables. Several demographic variables were included in analyses to control for their anticipated associations with outcome variables. Gender was dummy coded (male = 0, female = 1). Respondents were asked to identify their racial/ethnic status from a list that included *American Indian, Asian American or Pacific Islander, Black/African-American, Bi-racial, Hispanic-American, White/European-American,* and *other.* All respondents reported being either Black or White so the racial variable was dummy coded (Black = 0, White = 1). Respondents were asked to report their marital status as either *married, divorced, separated, widowed,* or *single/never married.* This variable was dummy coded (married = 1, all others = 0). Age was assessed by asking respondents what year they were born. Educational status was assessed with a one item ordinal measure that asked respondents to indicate the highest level of education that they had completed. The six-point response format ranged from *8th grade or less* (1) to *post-graduate work or graduate degree* (6). Household income was assessed with a one item ordinal measure. The nine-point response format ranged from *less than $10,000* (1) to *$80,000 or more* (9). Finally, employment status was assessed by asking respondents to indicate whether or not they were currently employed at the time of survey completion (yes/no format). Respondents who replied negatively were assigned a value of zero and those who responded positively were assigned a value of one.

RESULTS

Data were analyzed using hierarchical multiple regression. Entry of the variables proceeded in the following order: demographic control variables, caregiver stress, social support, and interaction terms between caregiver stress and each social support variable. Following guidelines by Aiken and West (1991), interaction terms were created by centering caregiver stress and social support variables to reduce potential problems with multicollinearity. Significant interaction terms were probed using simple slope analysis. High and low values on social support were represented respectively by one standard deviation above and below the centered mean of zero. Reported findings are those that are significant at the .05 level.

Bivariate associations among demographic variables, caregiver stress, social support variables, and indicators of grandparent psychological well-being are presented in Table 1. Marital status was associated positively but weakly with life satisfaction (.19, $p < .05$). Both educational status and household income were associated positively but weakly with generativity (.19, $p < .05$). Caregiver stress was associated negatively with both life satisfaction ($-.52$, $p < .01$) and generativity ($-.34$, $p < .01$). With the exception of enacted informal social support, each of the social support variables was associated positively with life satisfaction. All five of the social support variables were associated positively with generativity. Strongest associations were evident between perceived informal social support and life satisfaction (.39, $p < .01$) and between informal social support network and generativity (.42, $p < .01$).

As a preliminary step, we also examined whether several grandchild characteristics were related to caregiver stress, grandparent life satisfaction and generativity. These characteristics included age of grandchild, length of time grandchild has been in grandparent's custody, and number of grandchildren being raised. Correlational analysis revealed no significant associations between child-related factors and grandparent caregiver stress and outcome variables.

Regression analyses were undertaken to examine associations among caregiver stress, social support variables, life satisfaction, and generativity. Only those control variables and social support variables that emerged as statistically significant in the correlational analysis were included in regression models. This modeling approach was used to maximize statistical power (McClelland & Judd, 1993) and to ensure a more parsimonious set of models by including variables that are most relevant to the particular outcomes under consideration.

Table 2 summarizes findings from an analysis regressing life satisfaction on marital status, caregiver stress, social support variables, and stress-support interaction terms. Marital status was a significant predictor of life satisfaction (Beta = .19, $p < .05$), accounting for 4% of variance in this outcome measure. Marital status remained statistically

TABLE 1. Bivariate Associations Among Demographic Variables, Caregiver Stress, Social Support Variables, and Grandparent Psychological Well-Being

Variable	(1)	(2)	(3)	(4)	(5)	(6)	(7)	(8)	(9)	(10)	(11)	(12)	(13)	(14)	(15)
(1) Gender															
(2) Race	-.10														
(3) Marital status	-.14	.29**													
(4) Age	-.16	-.04	-.06												
(5) Education	.02	.12	.00	-.22*											
(6) Household income	-.12	.27	.63**	-.18*	.24**										
(7) Employment status	-.03	.07	-.01	-.25**	.20*	.26**									
(8) Caregiver stress	-.08	.01	-.04	-.07	.03	-.01	.07								
(9) Informal support network	.19*	-.08	.16	-.00	.02	.21*	-.05	-.27**							
(10) Perceived informal social support	.12	.01	.33	-.06	-.01	.24**	-.04	-.38**	.53**						
(11) Enacted informal social support	.15	.10	.11	-.11	.06	.14	-.04	-.18	.32**	.32**					
(12) Perceived formal social support	.14	.14	-.04	.08	.09	.00	-.19*	-.20*	-.01	.03	-.11				
(13) Enacted formal social support	.09	.03	-.14	.25**	.13	-.31**	-.25**	-.01	-.04	.02	-.13	.25**			
(14) Life satisfaction	.07	.02	.19*	.15	.10	.13	-.08	-.52**	.27*	.39**	.13	.22*	.23*		
(15) Generativity	.16	-.08	.06	.05	.19*	.19*	-.16	-.34**	.42**	.30**	.25**	.27**	.21*	.46**	
M	NA	NA	NA	NA	NA	NA	NA	2.30	25.72	5.5	5.54	3.48	.73	9.81	2.78
SD	NA	NA	NA	NA	NA	NA	NA	.62	6.09	7.48	1.11	.51	.35	4.63	.43

*Correlation is significant at the .05 level (t-tailed)
**Correlation is significant at the .01 level (t-tailed)

TABLE 2. Grandparent Life Satisfaction Regressed on Caregiver Stress and Social Support Variables ($N = 132$)

Independent Variables	Standardized Beta Coefficients			
	Block 1	Block 2	Block 3	Block 4
Marital status	.19*	.16*	.15*	.15*
Caregiver stress		−.51***	−.42***	−.42***
Informal support network			.07	.09
Perceived informal social support			.14	.15
Perceived formal social support			.08	.08
Enacted formal social support			.22**	.20**
Caregiver stress x informal support network				−.03
Caregiver stress x perceived informal support				.01
Caregiver stress x perceived formal support				.11
Caregiver stress x enacted formal support				−.01
$R^2\Delta$	.04*	.26***	.09***	.01
$F\Delta$	4.73*	47.97***	4.72***	.56
df	(1,131)	(1,130)	(4,126)	(4,122)
R^2	.04	.30	.39	.40
F	4.72***	27.19***	13.25***	8.07***
df1, df2	(1,131)	(2,130)	(6,126)	(10,122)

Note: * $p < .05$; ** $p < .01$; *** $p < .001$

significant after all variables were entered into the model; however, the beta coefficient attenuated slightly with the addition of caregiver stress and social support variables. As hypothesized, caregiver stress was associated negatively with life satisfaction (Beta = −.51, $p < .001$). As indicated in Block 2 of the table, caregiver stress accounted for 26% of variance in life satisfaction, but this reduced to 17% unique variance when social support variables were entered in Block 3 of the regression model. Social support variables accounted for an additional 9% of variance in life satisfaction. However, the only statistically significant main effect that emerged among the four social support variables was for enacted social support (Beta = .22, $p < .01$). None of the interaction terms between caregiver stress and social support were statistically significant. Thus, the hypothesis that social support buffers the association between caregiver stress and life satisfaction was not supported.

Table 3 summarizes findings from an analysis regressing generativity on demographic variables, caregiver stress, social support variables, and

TABLE 3. Grandparent Generativity Regressed on Caregiver Stress and Social Support Variables (*N* = 132)

Independent Variables	Standardized Beta Coefficients			
	Block 1	Block 2	Block 3	Block 4
Educational status	.15	.16	.10	.11
Household income	.15	.15	.16	.16
Caregiver stress		−.35***	−.21**	−.23**
Informal support network			.31***	.26**
Perceived informal social support			−.03	.06
Enacted informal social support			.14	.14
Perceived formal social support			.18*	.14
Enacted formal social support			.23**	.25*
Caregiver stress x informal support network				.08
Caregiver stress x perceived informal support				−.27**
Caregiver stress x enacted informal social support				.02
Caregiver stress x perceived formal support				.02
Caregiver stress x enacted formal support				−.02
$R^2\Delta$	.06	.12**	.20**	.05*
$F\Delta$	3.94*	18.74***	7.68***	1.99*
df	(2,130)	(1,129)	(5,124)	(5,119)
R^2	.06	.18	.37	.42
F	3.94*	9.23***	9.16***	6.56***
df	(2,130)	(3,129)	(8,124)	(13,119)

Note: † $p < .10$; * $p < .05$; ** $p < .01$; *** $p < .001$

stress-support interaction terms. The beta coefficients for educational status and household income did not reach the criterion for statistical significance (Beta for educational status = .15, $p > .05$; Beta for household income = .15, $p > .05$); however as a set, these variables accounted for a significant proportion of variance in generativity (6%). Caregiver stress was associated negatively and moderately with generativity (Beta = −.35, $p < .001$), accounting for 12% of variance. Social support variables accounted for an additional 20% of variance in generativity. Significant main effects were found for three of the five social support variables. These include informal support network (Beta = .31, $p = .001$), perceived formal social support (Beta = .18, $p < .05$), and enacted formal social support (Beta = .23, $p < .01$). The main effect for enacted informal social support was marginally significant (Beta = .14, p = .07). The positive beta coefficients indicate that higher levels of social support are related to a greater sense of generativity.

A main effect for perceived informal support did not emerge in this analysis. However, the interaction between caregiver stress and perceived informal social support was statistically significant (Beta = –.26, p < .01). Contrary to our hypothesis, perceived informal social support exacerbated the negative association between caregiver stress and generativity. The association between caregiver stress and generativity was significantly stronger for grandparents who perceived a high amount of informal social support (b = –.37, p < .001) compared to grandparents who perceived a low amount of informal social support (b = –.03, *ns.*)

DISCUSSION

This study examined the theoretical assumption that social support buffers the association between grandparent caregiver stress and both life satisfaction and generativity. The bivariate analysis indicated that caregiver stress is associated negatively with life satisfaction and generativity. Negative outcomes of stress have been well-documented in the caregiving literature. This association was further supported with these results. Informal and formal social support had a beneficial influence on stress outcomes regardless of the amount of stress participants experienced influencing the stress outcomes. Similar to recent caregiving investigations the moderating effect of social support was not found (Chappell & Reid, 2002; Miller et al., 2001). The informal and formal social support constructs used in this study did not present evidence that these dimensions of social support moderated the stress of raising a grandchild.

In the life satisfaction model, 40% of the variance was explained by marital status, caregiver stress, and enacted formal support. Often a marital partner is a key person in a support network. In our sample, slightly over half of the participants were married which is similar to national samples of grandparent caregivers (Fuller-Thomson, Minkler, & Driver, 1997). Perhaps the presence of a partner helped to alleviate the financial and household burdens associated with parenting. Caregiver stress was a robust predictor of life satisfaction, accounting for 17% of unique variance in this outcome measure. The negative relationship between caregiver stress and life satisfaction was expected as stress often impacts one's evaluation of life. Enacted formal support or the receipt of social services also appeared to be an important factor related to life satisfaction among grandparents raising grandchildren. This finding supports other research that grandparent caregivers utilize social services, especially services that involve other grandparent-grandchild family structures (Landry-Meyer, 1999b). Grandparents may feel more positive about life when receiving formal support specific to their needs.

Social support did not buffer the association between caregiver stress and life satisfaction. A possible explanation may be found in Cohen and Wills' (1985) review of the stress-buffering hypothesis. They suggest that for social support to be an effective moderator, there must be a match between the source of stress and the type of support. For instance, if a grandparent caregiver's source of stress is lack of child care, then child care support would be an effective resource and buffer the stress association. While various types of support were measured in this study, a global measure of caregiver stress was utilized.

In the generativity model, educational status, household income, caregiver stress, and social support variables accounted for 42% of variance in generativity. Social support variables accounted for 20% of the variation in generativity, primarily through perceived formal social support, enacted formal social support, and the informal support network of grandparents. With close to 19% of participants not graduating from high school and about one-third having annual incomes less than $19,000, the value of social services becomes critical to the nurturing of the next generation. This finding also lends support to grandparent caregivers' perceived need for social services to provide generational continuity when they can no longer rely on support once received from informal support network (Crowther & Rodriquez, 2003).

The informal support network accounted for approximately 10% of the unique variance in the generativity model. The network did not moderate the association between stress and generativity, suggesting that general benefits are derived from being embedded in a system of caring others regardless of the level of caregiving stress experienced by grandparent caregivers. According to Erikson (1963), this network or radius of significant others pressures individuals to resolve a psychosocial task, in this case, generativity. Life-stage-related demands are communicated to individuals through the network. Contrary to our expectations of a buffering influence and seemingly at odds with the positive influence of the informal support network on grandparents' sense of generativity, perceived informal social support acted as a detriment to the grandparent caregiver's achievement of generativity among those who reported a high degree of caregiver stress. Thus, while it may be that network members provide needed support to grandparents, they may also be a constant reminder that grandparent caregivers are off-time with same-age peers. Connections with friends and family who are engaged in on-time and better-rewarded paths to generativity may lead grandparent caregivers to feel like their contribution to society is less important especially with the increased stress associated with re-parenting. This perception would be even more likely if support network members are achieving a sense of generativity through work or creative endeavors (Kotre, 1984), for which a grandparent caregiver has no time. If a grandparent's support network is not engaged in similar life tasks or does not see re-parenting tasks as generative, then the grandparent caregiver might not perceive this support as helpful. With the use of generativity as a stress outcome, this research provides valuable insight into the individual developmental needs of grandparent caregivers.

In light of this finding, future research should distinguish between the effect of informal support networks among fellow grandparents raising grandchildren and the effect of informal support networks in which members have different life stage experiences. Because of the heterogeneity of life experiences, it is important to determine the impact of assuming an off-time role in one's individual development. The need to adapt standardized measures for use with this sub-population of grandparent caregivers in order to adequately identify and analyze the processes that contribute to feelings of generativity and life satisfaction are needed. In addition, research should measure specific stressors and match the stressor to type of support. While this study examined five types of social support and utilized a revised version of the Parenting Stress Index, future research should match specific stressors to type of support to determine the functional role of support in a grandparent caregiver's well-being.

It is important to note the possibility of gender differences in social support processes. Unfortunately, our sample makeup did not permit a test to determine whether our theoretical model differed for male and female grandparents because of the overrepresentation of female grandparents. However, bivariate analysis indicated minimal influence of gender on caregiver stress, social support variables, and outcome measures. Furthermore, follow-up regression analyses were conducted by dropping male grandparents from the sample and testing the theoretical model on female grandparents only to assess the extent to which gender influenced reported findings. Results from this set of analysis were highly similar to the full sample, and substantive findings were essentially unchanged.

This study builds on extant literature in three ways. First, although considerable theoretical attention has focused on the moderator effect of social support in the stress-adjustment relationship, few direct tests of the buffering hypothesis are evident in the literature on grandparent caregivers. Second, several dimensions of social support were tested. Research has shown that the benefits of social support to the individual vary depending on the type of social support that is assessed and the context in which it is assessed, such as the study population and the particular type of stressor paired with social support. Currently, little is known about how stressors and social support interact to shape the unique experience of grandparents raising grandchildren. Thus, to increase the precision of this inquiry, several types of social support measures were used to identify dimensions that are most salient in counteracting caregiving stress. And, finally, the family stress model was examined across two distinct stress outcome indicators–life satisfaction and generativity.

There are several study limitations. First, the study used a non-probability convenience sample. The participants may not represent the generalized population. Second, social support as an adaptation resource is a process. The study measured social support at one point in time rather than over a period of time. Third, the measure of the stressor represents a metaconstruct with a focus on re-parenting.

CONCLUSION AND IMPLICATIONS

Grandparents cope with the life course transition of becoming a surrogate parent to a grandchild. While social support was not found to moderate the association between caregiving stress and stress outcomes, regression analyses demonstrated that caregiver stress is associated negatively with life satisfaction and generativity. Practice and policy implications should focus on this association in supporting the grandparent-grandchild family structure. Decreasing caregiver stress appears to be critically important to the well-being of grandparent caregivers (Kelley et al., 2000). Intervention strategies guided by family stress theory can provide resources for grandparent caregivers as they adapt to the re-parenting role. For instance, the positive association between enacted formal social support and life satisfaction and generativity suggest that social service delivery systems can have a positive impact on grandparent-grandchild family structures.

Informal social network density was associated positively with generativity, after controlling for the influence of caregiver stress indicates the importance of a network of support in adult development. Given the association of marital status in predicting life satisfaction, practitioners should note the beneficial effect of a support network in raising a grandchild. In cases where the grandparent is single, practitioners should note the absence of co-resident network member and the potential need of a single grandparent to seek additional support. However, caution should be exercised in drawing definitive conclusions about the role of marital status in life satisfaction as this association is weak.

In order for social support to be an effective moderator of stress, the support must match the specificity of the stress. Specific social service programs geared to the unique stressors of raising a grandchild may prove more beneficial to grandparents raising grandchildren than generalized parent programs. For instance, Ohio has implemented the use of kinship navigators based on a statewide survey of specific service needs of grandparent caregivers (see Landry-Meyer, 1999b). These navigators assist grandparent caregivers with resource and referral specific to their caregiver stress. Social support programs should examine the functional role of social support in the caregiving context to best meet the needs of grandparent caregivers.

REFERENCES

Aiken, L. S., & West, S. G. (1991). *Multiple regression: Testing and interpreting interactions.* Newbury Park, CA: Sage Publications.

Barrera, M. (1986). Distinctions between social support concepts, measures, and models. *American Journal of Community Psychology, 14, (4),* 413-445.

Berry, J. O., & Jones, W. H. (1995). The parental stress scale: Initial psychometric evidence. *Journal of Social and Personal Relationships, 12,* 463-472.

Burton, L. M. (1992). Black grandparents rearing children of drug-addicted parents: Stressors, outcomes, and social service needs. *The Gerontologist, 32,* 744-751.

Caputo, R. K. (2000). Depression and health among grandmothers co-residing with grandchildren in two cohorts of women. *Families in Society: The Journal of Contemporary Human Services, 82,* 473-483.

Chappell, N. L., & Reid, R. C. (2002). Burden and well-being among caregivers: Examining the distinction. *The Gerontologist, 42,* 772-780.

Cohen, S., & Wills, T. A. (1985). Stress, social support, and the buffering hypothesis. *Psychological Bulletin, 98,* 310-335.

Crowther, M., & Rodriguez, R. (2003). A stress and coping model of custodial grandparents among African Americans. In B. Hayslip, Jr. & J. H. Patrick (Eds.), *Working with custodial grandparents* (pp. 145-162). NY: Springer Publishing Co.

Downey, K. (1998). *Project report for grandparents raising grandchildren task force, State of Ohio.* Cincinnati, OH: Institute for Policy Research, University of Cincinnati.

Erikson, E. H. (1963). *Childhood and society, 2nd edition.* NY: Norton.

Fisher, B. J. (1995). Successful aging, life satisfaction, and generativity in later life. *International Journal of Aging and Human Development, 41,* 239-250.

Fuller-Thomson, E., Minkler, M., & Driver, D. (1997). A profile of grandparents raising grandchildren in the United States. *The Gerontologist, 37,* 406-411.

Fuller-Thomson, E., & Minkler, M. (2000). The mental and physical health of grandmothers who are raising their grandchildren. *Journal of Mental Health and Aging, 6,* 311-323.

Giarusso, R., Feng, D., Silverstein, M., & Marenco, A. (2000). Primary and secondary stressors of grandparents raising grandchildren: Evidence from a national survey. *Journal of Mental Health and Aging, 6,* 291-310.

Hill, R. (1949). *Families under stress.* Westport, CT: Greenwood.

Jendrek, M. P. (1993). Grandparents who parent their grandchildren: Effects on life-style. *Journal of Marriage and the Family, 55,* 609-621.

Kelley, S. J., Whitley, D., Sipe, T. A., & Yorker, B. C. (2000). Psychological distress in grandmother kinship care providers: The role of resources, social support, and physical health. *Child Abuse and Neglect, 24,* 311-321.

Kotre, J. (1984). *Outliving the self: How we live on in the future generations.* MA: Johns Hopkins Press.

Lai, D. Attitude Toward Use of Formal Services. (personal communication, October 15, 1996).

Landry-Meyer, L. (1999a). Grandparents raising grandchildren: An investigation of roles and support. (Doctoral dissertation, The Ohio State University). *Dissertation Abstracts* (UMI No. 072699)

Landry-Meyer, L. (1999b). Research into action: Recommendations and intervention strategies for grandparent caregivers. *Family Relations, 48,* 381-391.

Landry-Meyer, L., & Newman, B. M. (in press). Grandparent caregivers: An exploration of roles. *Journal of Family Issues.*

Litwak, E. (1985). *Helping the elderly: The complementary roles of informal networks and formal systems.* New York: Guilford Press.

Lubben, J. E. (1988). Assessing social networks among elderly population. *Family and Community Health, 11,* 42-52.

McAdams, D. P., & de St. Aubin, E. (1992). A theory of generativity and its assessment through self-report, behavioral acts, and narrative themes in autobiography. *Journal of Personality and Social Psychology, 62,* 1003-1015.

McClelland, G. H., & Judd, C. M. (1993). Statistical difficulties of detecting interactions and moderator effects. *Psychological Bulletin, 114,* 376-390.

Miller, B., Townsend, A., Carpenter, E., Montgomery, R. V. J., Stull, D., & Young, R. F. (2001). Social support and caregiver distress. *Journal of Gerontology: Social Sciences, 56B,* S249-S256.

Minkler, M., Roe, K. M., & Robertson-Beckley, R. J. (1994). Raising children from crack-cocaine households: Effects on family and friendship ties of African American women. *American Journal of Orthopsychiatry, 64,* 20-29.

Neugarten, B., Havighurst, R. J., & Tobin, S. S. (1961). The measurement of life satisfaction. *Journal of Gerontology, 16,* 134-143.

Pearlin, L. I., Mullan, J. T., Semple, S. J., & Skaff, M. M. (1990). Caregiving and the stress process: An overview of concepts and their comments. *The Gerontologist, 30,* 583-594.

Roberto, K. A., & Qualls, S. H. (2003). Intervention strategies for grandparents raising grandchildren: Lessons learned from the caregiving literature. In B. Hayslip, Jr. & J. H. Patrick (Eds.), *Working with custodial grandparents* (pp. 13-26). NY: Springer.

Saluter, A. F. (1992). *Marital status and living arrangements: Current population reports, population characteristics. Series P-20, No. 461.* Washington, DC: U.S. Government Printing Office.

Sands, R. G., & Goldberg-Glen, R. S. (2000). Factors associated with stress among grandparents raising grandchildren. *Family Relations, 49,* 97-105.

Strawbridge, W. J., Wallhagen, M. I., & Cohen, R. D. (2002). Successful aging and well-being: Self-rated compared with Rowe and Kahn. *The Gerontologist, 42,* 727-733.

Vaux, A. & Harrison, D. (1985). Support network characteristics associated with support Satisfaction and perceived support. *American Journal of Community Psychology, 13,* 245-268.

Zimet, G. D., Dahlmen, N. W., Zimet, S. G., & Farley, G. K. (1988). The Multidimensional Scale of Perceived Social Support. *Journal of Personality Assessment, 52,* 30-41.

Skipped Generation Families:
Sources of Psychological Distress Among Grandmothers of Grandchildren Who Live in Homes Where Neither Parent Is Present

Terry L. Mills
Zenta Gomez-Smith
Jessica M. De Leon

SUMMARY. Today, more than at any period in U.S. history, more grandparents are raising their grandchildren. In many instances, the biological parents are absent from these grandparent-headed households for a variety of reasons. Although grandfathers and grandmothers both serve in the role of surrogate parents, grandparent caregiving can be seen as a "women's issue" when examined from the broader sociological context of gender. Using data from the National Survey of America's Families, this study examined factors associated with the frequency of

Terry L. Mills is Associate Professor, University of Florida, Department of Sociology. Zenta Gomez-Smith is a doctoral student, University of Florida, Department of Sociology, 3219 Turlington Hall, Gainesville, FL 32611-7330. Jessica M. De Leon is Coordinator, Research Program Services, University of Florida College of Pharmacy, Pharmacy Health Care Administration, Gainesville, FL 32610-0496.

Address correspondence to: Terry L. Mills, University of Florida, Department of Sociology, 3219 Turlington Hall, Gainesville, FL 32611-7330 (E-mail: tlmills@soc.ufl.edu).

[Haworth co-indexing entry note]: "Skipped Generation Families: Sources of Psychological Distress Among Grandmothers of Grandchildren Who Live in Homes Where Neither Parent Is Present." Mills, Terry L., Zenta Gomez-Smith, and Jessica M. De Leon. Co-published simultaneously in *Marriage & Family Review* (The Haworth Press, Inc.) Vol. 37, No. 1/2, 2005, pp. 191-212; and: *Challenges of Aging on U.S. Families: Policy and Practice Implications* (ed: Richard K. Caputo.) The Haworth Press, Inc., 2005, pp. 191-212. Single or multiple copies of this article are available for a fee from The Haworth Document Delivery Service [1-800-HAWORTH, 9:00 a.m. - 5:00 p.m. (EST). E-mail address: docdelivery@haworthpress.com].

feelings of psychosocial distress among grandmother caregivers of grandchildren in skipped generation families. Multivariate regression models indicate that for these grandmothers, being Black and living in the Midwest, having a family income below the poverty level, having Medicaid or SCHIP coverage, not receiving Welfare payments for childcare, and having a usual place for health care were all associated with more frequent feelings of psychosocial distress. On the other hand, being married, receiving social services help with childcare, grandmother's perception of less parenting burden, and living below poverty in the Midwest were associated with less frequent feelings of psychosocial distress. *[Article copies available for a fee from The Haworth Document Delivery Service: 1-800-HAWORTH. E-mail address: <docdelivery@haworthpress.com> Website: <http://www.HaworthPress.com> © 2005 by The Haworth Press, Inc. All rights reserved.]*

KEYWORDS. Skipped generation families, grandparent caregivers, surrogate parenting, psychosocial distress, depression, intergenerational co-residency

U.S. Census reports indicate that nearly 5.5 million children under age 18 co-reside in homes with a grandparent. This number represents about 7.7% of all children under age 18 in the United States (U.S. Census, 1999, 2000). Further, about 1.3 million of these children live in grandparent-headed households where neither parent is present (Bryson & Casper, 1999); and roughly half of the grandchildren in such families are under age 6 (U.S. Census, 1999).

It is not a new phenomenon for a grandparent to intervene or assist in raising their grandchildren or other relatives (Mills, 2001). Rather, what is new is the dramatic increase in this phenomenon. For example, Bryson and Casper (1999) reported that between 1992 and 1997, the greatest growth in intergenerational co-residence occurred among grandchildren living with grandparents with no parent present. Goodman and Silverstein (2001) reported that although most grandparent-headed households provide for the grandchild and one or both parents, approximately 36% have neither parent living in the home, implying that the grandparents have complete responsibility for the care of the grandchild.

Fuller-Thompson, Minkler, and Driver (1997) have referred to grandparent-headed households where neither parent is present as, "skipped generation" families. These skipped generation families have increased as a consequence of several social problems including: the increase in drug abuse, teen pregnancy, divorce and the rapid rise of single-parent households, mental and physical illness, AIDS, crime, child abuse and neglect, and incarceration of parents (Bryson & Casper, 1999). The increase in the number of grandchildren and grandparents who co-reside reflects sociodemographic characteristics of the grandparents and their progeny, as well as contemporary social problems (Caputo, 2001).

The purpose of this study was to examine skipped generation households to determine the context wherein grandmother caregivers of grandchildren experience psychosocial distress. Specifically, the study was concerned with the effects of the sociodemographic characteristics of the grandmother and grandchild, factors associated with the grandmother's social support, the grandchild's physical health and access to health care; and the grandmother's perceived parental burden. An advantage of this study is that the data are from a national probability sample, which allows us to make inferences about the U.S. population.

BACKGROUND

The Psychological Status of Grandparent Caregivers

Pruchno and McKenney (2002) examined the psychological well-being of 867 Black and White grandmothers (aged 50-83 yrs) caring for children (aged 5-18 yrs) in the absence of the child's parents. They reported that both positive and negative affect was predicted by grandparent's health and caregiver burden. In particular, caregiving satisfaction was a unique predictor of positive affect, while grandchild behavior was a unique predictor of negative affect. Poor physical health and feelings of caregiving burden increased negative affect and decreased positive feelings.

Other research has looked at caregiver grandparents' stress in contrast to parental stress. Harrison, Richman, and Vittimberga (2000) used a sample consisting of the caregivers for 82 children with behavioral problems. They grouped the sample into grandparent (n = 18), single parent (n = 49), and two-parent (n = 15) families. They found that grandparents reported experiencing less stress than the other two family groups, and found no statistically significant differences between single-parent families and two-parent families. However, the results may have been affected by the differences in sizes of the groups, and a generally small sample overall. Also, the results may have been affected by the sampling procedure, which used families referred to an outpatient child and family therapy clinic.

Empirical studies have also examined the effects of the relationships between grandmother, parents, and grandchildren on the life satisfaction and well-being of the caregiver grandmother (Goodman & Silverstein, 2001). This research found that the strength and existence of the intergenerational relationships do affect the life satisfaction of the parenting grandmother. Those grandmothers who had strong relations with both the parent of the child and the grandchild, and who themselves acted as a mediator for the family, had greater life satisfaction and well-being in other arrangements of intergenerational relationships.

Minkler and Fuller-Thompson (1999) analyzed grandparents who are caregivers compared to grandparents who are not caregivers. They used measures of ADL (activities of daily living), which considers both physical and mental limitations, and found significant differences of ADL between the two types of grandparents. For instance, parenting grandparents were less satisfied with their health than non-parenting grandparents. They also found that parenting grandparents have higher odds of experiencing ADL limitations. Minkler and Fuller-Thompson (1997) note that these findings are consistent with their previous research that found higher depression in parenting grandparents than in non-parenting grandparents.

In a 1996 study, Giarrusso, Feng, Wang, and Silverstein compared the well-being and family solidarity of parenting grandparents, co-parenting grandparents, and non-parenting grandparents. They used data from 659 grandparents who were involved in at least two successive waves of the USC Longitudinal Study of Generations. They found that grandparents who are involved in parenting their grandchildren, either parenting or co-parenting, are more likely to be younger and have poorer health than grandparents who do not parent. Giarrusso and colleagues also found that parenting grandparents experience more feelings of family obligation than both co-parenting and non-parenting grandparents. In terms of psychological well-being, co-parenting grandparents were found to do better than parenting grandparents.

Racial Distinctions Among Grandparent Caregivers

Research by Sands and Goldberg-Glen (2000) considered Black and White grandparents' well-being in terms of psychological stress and anxiety. Their sample consisted of 129 grandparents who were the primary caregivers of one or more of their grandchildren. They found that younger grandparents experienced higher levels of psychological stress and anxiety. Also, their findings suggested that those grandparents who cared for grandchildren with psychological and/or physical problems, as well as the grandparents who had a shortage of family cohesion were most likely to experience stress and anxiety.

Goodman and Silverstein (2001) found that compared to grandmothers of other ethnic groups, African American grandmothers were more likely to have more life satisfaction and lower negative affect. However, further empirical research has pointed to other reasons that suggest the issue of grandparents as caregivers for their grandchildren is especially relevant for African Americans. In the United States, the largest percentages of children living in a grandparent headed household are African American (Pebley & Rudkin, 1999; Pinson-Millburn & Fabian, 1996; Fuller-Thompson & Minkler, 2000; Caputo, 2001). Studies have found that compared to White grandparents who are caregivers to their grandchildren, African American parenting grandparents are more likely to be unemployed, live below the poverty line, and have more grandchildren for whom they provide care (Sands & Goldberg-Glen, 2000). Similarly, others have found that living beneath the poverty line, being African American, and being single raises the probability of becoming a grandparent who is a caregiver to their grandchildren (Roe & Minkler, 1998).

Fuller-Thompson and Minkler (2000) looked at African American grandparents' physical and mental health, and focused on the differences between those grandparents who parent their grandchildren and those who do not. They reported that African American grandparents who were caregivers were more likely to be female, have more grandchildren, and live below the poverty line than African American grandparents who were not caregivers. In terms of physical and mental health, caregiver grandparents had more ADL (activities of daily living) limitations and more symptoms of depression than African American grandparents who were not caregivers.

While grandparents as caregivers are most prevalent in African American families, the phenomenon is not limited to any racial or ethic population (Fuller-Thompson & Minkler, 2000; Pinson-Millburn & Fabian, 1996). The experiences and expectations may vary through ethnic groups (Pinson-Millburn & Fabian, 1996), and the empirical research on custodial grandparents has recently begun to explore other racial and ethnic minority groups (Burnette, 1999). A related study by Caputo

(2001) found that among coresident households with young grandmothers race was nonsignificant as a predictor of coresidence. He suggested that many of the factors associated with grandchildren residing with grandparents are located more in urban areas where there is a higher incidence of social problems.

Family Structure and Welfare Entry Among Children Living with Grandparents

Family structure is central to understanding differences in economic disadvantage and welfare entries of grandchildren in grandparent-headed households. Evidence suggests that welfare use among skipped generation households is disproportionately high (Chalfie, 1994; Fuller-Thompson, Minkler, & Driver, 1997). It has been suggested that entering into welfare hinges on the resources available to grandparents when grandchildren move into their homes (Brandon, 2000). The family adaptation literature and family stress theory suggest that families adapt when confronted with increased pressures on limited resources, like providing for an additional dependent (Sorensen & McLanahan, 1990). Adaptations can include increasing labor supply, cutting back on expenses, moving to cheaper housing, or going into welfare. It is established that the poverty rates among grandchildren in grandparent's households are higher than among children living with two parents (Brandon, 2000).

A Profile of Grandchildren Living with Their Grandparents

Grandparents are being called upon to raise grandchildren of all ages. The largest group of children (51% in 1998) is preschoolers or under age six years old, while 49% are between age 6 through 17 (National Committee to Preserve Social Security and Medicare, 1998). Grandchildren raised by grandparents often suffer from emotional and behavioral problems due to prior abuse, neglect, and abandonment (Kelly, Yorker, & Whitley, 1997). Grandchildren in grandmother only, no parent present households are most likely to be poor and to have received public assistance (Casper & Bryson, 1998).

Children's Access to Health Care

Having adequate access to health care can significantly influence care use and health outcomes. Even where health care services are readily available, people may not have a usual source of health care or may experience barriers to receiving services because of financial or insurance restrictions, a lack of availability of providers at night or on weekends, or other difficulties. Data indicate that Black children are less likely than White children to have a usual source of health care. Among children under age 18 who had a usual source of care, about 41% had a provider who did not have night and weekend office hours. Additionally, 22% of these children's families found their usual source of care providers "somewhat" or "Very" difficult to contact by telephone (Weigers, Weinick, & Cohen, 1998). Consequently, barriers to a grandchild's access to health care may very well be associated with the grandmother's psychosocial distress, particularly if the child has fair or poor health.

Assessment of the Relevant Literature

Much of the previous research on the psychological well-being of caregiving grandparents have been comparative studies that examined the sources of stress of non-caregiving grandparents versus caregiving grandparents; or caregiving grandparents versus parents. Moreover, these prior studies have primarily emphasized the effect on psychological distress of the grandparent re-entering the parental role, the grandparent's perception of caregiver burden, the grandparent's health status, or the quality of the relationship with the parents. However, there is a dearth of empirical studies that have explicitly conducted within-group analyses of the factors associated with psychosocial distress among grandmothers in skipped generation households. For example, little is known about how the demographic or health/behavioral factors of the grandchild are related to the skipped generation grandmothers' psychosocial distress. Additionally, there are not many studies that have investigated whether the variance in the frequency of psychosocial distress among skipped generation grandmothers is associated with their own demographic characteristics, or the context of their social support. Finally, only a few previous studies of grandparent caregivers have employed national probability samples. Based upon a review of the relevant literature and our interest expanding our understanding of the factors associated with the psychosocial distress of grandmothers in skipped generation households, we investigated the following research questions:

1. Does the grandchild's race, sex, or age influence the grandmother's frequency of feeling psychosocial distress?

2. Does the grandmother's race, sex, or age, affect the frequency of feelings of psychosocial distress?
3. What factors associated with the grandmother's social support are related to the frequency of psychosocial distress?
4. In what ways does the grandchild's physical health and access to health care influence the occurrence of the grandmother's psychosocial distress?

METHOD

The Data

The data for the present study are from the 1999 wave of the National Survey of America's Families that is designed to produce estimates that are representative of the civilian, noninstitutionalized population under age 65. In order to reduce respondent burden, a decision was made to subsample household members. If there were multiple children under age 6, one was randomly selected (Focal child #1). The same was done for children ages 6 to 17 (Focal child #2). No more than two children were sampled from each household. Data were collected about each of these sample children through the most knowledgeable adult (MKA) in the household for that child. In choosing the MKA, interviewers asked to speak to the person in the household who knew the most about the sampled child's education and health care. In families with two sampled children, the MKA was not necessarily the same person for both children. Consequently, there were cases in which one family had two MKAs (NSAF, 1999a).

The NSAF draws households from two separate sampling frames. The first frame consists of households from a random-digit dial (RDD) sample of households with telephones. However, because households without telephone service contain a disproportionate number of low-income children, a supplementary area sample was conducted in person for those households without telephones. The area sample provides data for these and other families without current phone service.

Oversize samples were drawn in 13 states (Alabama, California, Colorado, Florida, Massachusetts, Michigan, Minnesota, Mississippi, New Jersey, New York, Texas, Washington, and Wisconsin) to allow the production of reliable estimates at the state level. Further, the oversize state samples were supplemented with a balance of the U.S. sample to allow the creation of estimates at the national level as well.

The Subsample

The analytic subsample was constructed to include only MKAs who were the grandmothers of grandchildren living in households where neither parent was present. This inclusion criterion resulted in 165 primary sampling unit (PSU) observations that when weighted with the appropriate adult or child weights represent a population estimate of 430,018 grandmothers and 364,371 grandchildren. The child weights include factors that adjust for the probability of selecting the child (including differential factors by reported poverty level on the screener and the number of children per household), and nonresponse at the household and person level. Furthermore, the weights are adjusted to be consistent with known totals of the number of children by race, Hispanic ethnicity, age, sex, and tenure (renting or owning a home) for each study area and the nation. The adult weights were developed to produce estimates of all adults 18 to 64 years old, for most of the questions relevant to adults in the NSAF.

Data Analysis Procedures

Weighted descriptive and multivariate analyses were used to produce population frequency distributions and regression outputs. Because the NSAF is complex survey data, a decision was made to not use standard statistical software. Rather, for these analyses STATA™ was used to assure more accurate estimates of population parameters (Stata Statistical Software, n.d.). Point estimates of population parameters are impacted by the value of the analysis weight for each observation. Standard statistical software packages typically do not consider four common characteristics of sample survey data: (1) unequal probability selection of observation, (2) clustering of observations, (3) stratification, and (4) nonresponse and other adjustments (Brogan, 1998). We performed hierarchical multiple regression analysis with the grandmother's level of psychosocial distress as the dependent variable, and the grandchild's demographic characteristics, the grandmother's demographic characteristics, the grandmother's context of social support; a measure of the grandmother's parenting burden; and the grandchild's physical health status and access to health care as independent variables. These multivariate analyses used the STATA "svy" procedures that were developed to process survey data such as the NSAF.

Dependent Variable

An index of the grandmother's level of psychosocial distress was constructed using five items that asked the grandmother (MKA) how much of the time during the past month they: felt nervous, calm and peaceful, felt downhearted, was a happy person, or could not be cheered up. Each item was measured on a Likert-type scale that ranged from "All of the time" (1) to "None of the time" (4). The two positive items (felt calm and peaceful; and was a happy person) were reverse-coded. The scores for the psychosocial index ranged from 5-20, with *lower scores representing more frequent psychosocial distress.* Chronbach's alpha reliability coefficient for the psychosocial well-being index was .845, which indicates that the scale has sufficient homogeneity (Nunnally, 1978).

Independent Variables

Grandmother/Grandchild Demographic Factors. Race was coded as "Whites/Others" (0), and "Black" (1). Sex of the grandchild was coded as "Male" (0) and "Female" (1). Chronological age was a continuous variable. The grandmother's marital status variable asked whether the MKA has a spouse or unmarried partner; and was coded "No" (0) and "Yes" (1).

Grandmother's Social Support Factors. The number of relatives in the household was a continuous measure ranging from 0 to 15. Family income (for 1998) as a percent of poverty was initially operationalized as a categorical scale from "less than 50% below the poverty line" (0.5), to "equal or greater than 300% of poverty" (4). The poverty variable was recoded into a binary variable representing, "family income is < 50% to < 150% of poverty line" (e.g., severe poverty or near poor coded = 1), and "family income is 150% to 300% or greater than the poverty line" (e.g., above the poverty line coded = 0). Public agency help with childcare was operationalized with a question asking the MKA, "Did anyone from a foster care or social services agency help arrange for childcare?" This variable was coded "No" (0) and "Yes" (1). Welfare payment help with childcare was operationalized by asking, "does anyone in the household receive public assistance or welfare payments to help care for the child?" The welfare payment variable was coded "Yes" (0) and "No" (1). The grandmothers were asked whether any household member currently has Medicaid, SCHIP, or state coverage at the time of the interview. These three public programs were combined because the variables for each of the three different types of coverage were not designed for separate analysis (see NSAF, 1999b). The Medicaid/SCHIP variable was coded "No" (0) and "Yes" (1).

Grandchild's Physical Health Factors. The grandmother was asked whether the grandchild has any health condition that limits the child's activity. This was operationalized using the question, "Does (CHILD) have a physical, learning, or mental health condition that limits participation in the usual kinds of activities done by most children (his/her) age; or that limits ability to do regular school work?" The activity variable was coded "No" (0) and "Yes" (1). The grandchild's physical health status was assessed by the grandmother as either fair/poor (1), or "good, very good, or excellent" (0). The number of well child doctor visits during the past 12 months was a continuous measure ranging from 0-9. Also, the survey asked the grandmother whether the family had "a usual place for medical care?" This categorical variable was coded "No" (0) and "Yes" (1).

Grandmother's Parenting Burden. A parent burden index was constructed by summing the responses to four items that asked how often in the past month the MKA felt: the child was much harder to care for than most, felt the child did things that really bothered the MKA a lot, felt he or she was giving up more of his or her life to meet the child's needs than he or she ever expected, and felt angry with the child. The response categories included "All of the time" (coded 1), "Most of the time" (coded 2), "Some of the time" (coded 3), and "None of the time" (coded 4). Responses were totaled creating a scale score ranging from 4 to 16. Scores for respondents who answered three of the four questions were standardized to the 16-point scale. *Higher scores mean less parenting aggravation* (see NSAF, 1999b). Chronbach's alpha reliability coefficient for the parent burden scale was .70.

Geographic Regions. The data were categorized into four geographic regions: West, Midwest, Northeast, and South. A series of dummy variables were constructed to represent "All other regions" (0) and "West" (1); "All other regions" (0) and "South" (1); "All other regions" (0) and "Northeast" (1); "All other regions" (0) and "Midwest" (1). Because 38% of the grandmothers living in the South had family incomes below the poverty level, the South was included in the regression model. The geographic region with the next highest level of poverty among skipped generation households (18%) was the Midwest, so it was also included in the regression model.

RESULTS

Table 1 and Table 2 show the descriptive analyses of our data. About 69% of the grandmothers in our sample were Black, compared to 31% who were Whites and others. Approximately 6% of the grandmothers were classified as "other race." On the other hand, 62% of the grandchildren were Black, while 38% of the grandchildren were White or other. Three percent of the grandchildren were classified as "other race." The mean age of the grandchildren was 5.5 years (SD = 3.49), with an age range of between 0-16 years. Further, 66% of the grandchildren were under 6 years old, compared with 34% of the grandchildren who were between ages 6-16. The average age of the grandmothers was 51.1 years (SD = 7.15), with an age range of between 32-71 years.

A zero-order correlation matrix (available upon request) revealed that there were low correlations found between the dependent variable (level of psychosocial distress) and each of the independent variables. Further, we examined the bivariate relationship between the indepen-

TABLE 1. Descriptive Characteristics of Grandparents (N = 430,018–weighted)

	Proportion	Mean	SD	Range
Age	100%	51.1	7.15	32-71
Race				
Black	69%			
White/Other	31%			
Has spouse or partner	45%			
Number of relatives in household		3.8	1.40	2-15
Family income as % of poverty				
Below poverty levels	69%			
Above poverty levels	31%			
Receive welfare assistance	45%			
Yes	45%			
No	55%			
Currently has Medicaid/SCHIP/etc.	56%			
Received public support for childcare	21%			
Has usual place for health care	95%			
Psychosocial Well-Being Scale		14.53	3.22	5-20
Parent Burden Scale		12.05	2.99	6-16

TABLE 2. Descriptive Characteristics of Grandchildren (N = 364,370–weighted)

	Proportion	Mean	SD	Range
Age	100%	5.46	3.49	0-16
Focal child #1	61%	3.06	1.52	0-5
Focal child #2	39%	9.10	2.56	6-16
Gender				
Females	41%			
Males	59%			
Race				
Black	62%			
White/Other	38%			
Child has activity limitations	11%			
Number of well child visits		1.6	1.83	0-9
Health status				
Fair or poor health	6%			
Good or excellent health	94%			

dent variables to determine whether multicollinearity existed. The bivariate analysis indicated a modest association between whether any family member received welfare assistance and poverty level (–0.353; p < .0001); and whether any family member received welfare assistance and whether the family receives social service help with child care (–0.397; p < .0001).

In Table 3 we present four hierarchical models showing ordinary least squares regressions of grandmother's level of psychosocial distress on: (1) the grandmother's and grandchild's demographic factors; (2) adding factors associated with the grandmother's context of social support; (3) adding indicators of the grandchild's physical health and access to health care, whether the family had a usual source of health care; and an indicator of the grandmother's parenting burden; and (4) adding the main effect of geographic regions, and tests of interactions between level of poverty and region; and grandmother's race and region. In each model, standardized Beta coefficients are presented with standard error shown in parentheses.

As shown, in Model 1 the results revealed that when controlling for the grandmother's and grandchild's demographic factors, only the grandmother's age was significantly associated with the frequency of feelings of psychosocial distress. The results demonstrate that younger

TABLE 3. Regressions of Grandparents' Self-Reported Psychosocial Distress on Sociodemographic, Health, Behavioral, and Region

Variable	Model 1– Beta (SE)	Model 2– Beta (SE)	Model 3– Beta (SE)	Model 4– Beta (SE)
GChild race (Black = 1)	−2.44 (1.75)	−3.35 (1.66)*	−2.85 (2.45)	−1.85 (2.19)
GChild sex (Female = 1)	−0.02 (0.84)	−0.58 (0.87)	−0.93 (0.87)	0.02 (0.66)
GChild age	0.02 (0.09)	0.02 (0.10)	0.03 (0.09)	0.09 (0.09)
GP race (Black = 1)	1.61 (1.73)	−1.15 (0.76)	0.89 (2.53)	1.65 (2.23)
GP age	0.12 (0.04)**	0.05 (0.06)	0.05 (0.06)	−0.03 (0.05)
GP has spouse/partner	–	−1.12 (0.77)	1.77 (0.75)*	2.95 (0.66)***
# relatives in household	–	0.21 (0.23)	0.26 (0.17)	0.41 (0.17)**
Income below poverty level	–	−1.49 (1.17)	−1.54 (1.09)	−3.24 (0.77)***
Social service help with child care	–	3.61 (0.95)***	3.16 (0.85)***	2.24 (0.94)**
No welfare payment help for child	–	−1.42 (1.01)	−2.50 (0.99)**	−1.70 (0.98)
Has current Medicaid/SCHIP/etc.	–	−2.70 (1.13)**	−2.97 (1.08)**	−1.94 (.984)*
GChild has disability	–	–	.279 (.690)	.701 (.667)
GChild has fair/poor health	–	–	−.797 (1.29)	−.959 (1.15)
# of well child visits in past year	–	–	.096 (.211)	.121 (.192)
Have usual place for health care	–	–	−2.77 (.842)***	−2.35 (1.10)*
Parent burden level	–	–	.297 (.108)**	.261 (.093)*
Live in the Midwest	–	–	–	.976 (1.13)
(Race * Midwest)	–	–	–	−5.31 (1.36)***
(Poverty * Midwest)	–	–	–	6.99 (1.36)***
Constant	8.74 (2.28)***	12.80 (3.279)***	11.73 (3.46)***	16.12 (3.58)***
R^2	.109	.295	.383	.563

*** $p < .001$ ** $p < .01$ * $p < .05$

grandmothers reported psychosocial distress more frequently than older grandmothers ($\beta = -.122$).

In Model 2 when we included factors associated with the context of the grandmother's social support, the grandmother's age became nonsignificant. However, in this model the grandchild's race became significant ($\beta = -3.35$), such that having a Black grandchild was associated with more frequent occurrences of psychosocial distress, compared to if the grandchild was White. Further, this model also shows that currently receiving Medicaid or SCHIP assistance was significantly related to increased frequency of psychosocial distress ($\beta = -2.70$). Yet if the family received social services help with childcare the grandmother reported significantly fewer feelings of psychosocial distress ($\beta = 3.61$).

In Model 3 we included factors related to the grandchild's physical health and access to health care, whether the family had a usual place for health care, and an indicator of the grandmother's level of parenting burden. The results illustrate that when controlling for demographic and social support factors, several factors increased the frequency of the grandmother's feelings of psychosocial distress including: *not* receiving welfare assistance ($\beta = -2.50$), currently receiving Medicaid or SCHIP ($\beta = -2.97$), and having a usual place for health care ($\beta = -2.76$). On the other hand, being married ($\beta = 1.77$), receiving social service help with childcare ($\beta = 3.16$), and having a perception of lower parenting burden ($\beta = 0.30$) were significantly associated with grandmothers having less frequent feelings of psychosocial distress.

In Model 4 we included the effects of living in the South or Midwest, while controlling for the sociodemographic, social support, and health-related factors. When we accounted for the main effect of geographic region the results revealed that living below the poverty level ($\beta = -3.24$), receiving Medicaid or SCHIP ($\beta = -1.94$), and having a usual place for health care ($\beta = -2.35$) were all significantly associated with greater frequency of psychosocial distress among skipped generation grandmothers. Additionally, not receiving welfare payments for childcare approached significance as a factor contributing to the grandmother's more frequent feelings of psychosocial distress ($\beta = -1.70$, p = .08). Conversely, being married ($\beta = 2.95$), having other relatives living in the household ($\beta = 0.41$), receiving social services help with childcare ($\beta = 2.24$), and grandmother's perception of low-level of parenting burden ($\beta = 0.26$) were significantly related to less frequent feelings of psychosocial distress.

Additionally, we tested interactions between race and the two geographic regions; as well as poverty level when living in these geographic regions. There were no significant interactions related to living in the South. Yet, tests of interactions with the Midwest region show two important relationships. First, despite the overall negative affect of living below the poverty level, those grandmothers who were poor and lived in the Midwest reported fewer instances of psychosocial distress ($\beta = 6.99$), when compared to their counterparts in other geographic regions. Second, the interactions showed that race is a factor for Black grandmothers who live in the Midwest. The results indicated that these Black grandmothers reported more frequent ($\beta = -5.31$) occurrences of psychosocial distress than White grandmothers living in the Midwest, or Black and White grandmothers living in other regions of the United States. The geographic distribution showed that 14% of the Black skipped generation grandmothers lived in the Midwest, compared to 41% of their counterparts who lived in the South.

DISCUSSION

Grandparent caregivers face a myriad of challenges in nearly all aspects of their lives when they assume the role of parent. As a result, they are prone to psychological and emotional strain as well as feelings of helplessness and isolation. Often, grandparent caregivers neglect their own physical and emotional health because they give priority to the needs of their grandchildren. It has been argued that grandparent caregiving is largely a "women's issue" and that this gendered perspective can be viewed from a broader sociological context of caregiving vis-à-vis the ambivalent accounts of grandmothers raising their grandchildren as "silent saviors," while also being disparaged for their perceived failures as parents of their own children. Moreover, as a "women's issue" grandparent caregiving is a social problem that largely effects low-income women (Minkler, 1999).

The present study examined grandmother caregivers in skipped generation households to determine the ways that social factors such as gender, age, race, the context of the grandmother's social support, and the grandchild's health status or access to health care affect the frequency of psychosocial distress of grandmothers in skipped generation households. Several important associations emerged from our analyses.

When we accounted for the effects of the grandmother's and the grandchild's demographic characteristics we found that younger grandmothers were likely to experience psychosocial distress more frequently than their older counterparts. This finding is consistent with prior studies reporting that younger grandparents experienced higher levels of anxiety and psychological stress (Sands & Goldberg-Glen, 2000; Caputo, 2001). It has been suggested that younger grandparents are highly likely to experience psychological stress in trying to adjust to the demands of their own careers and personal interests (Caputo, 2001). However, in our study, the negative effect of being a younger grandparent was negated when we controlled for the effects of the grandmother's social support mechanisms. This suggests the importance of social assistance especially for younger grandmother caregivers, to help them to fulfill their own lives, while coping with the responsibilities of providing care for their grandchildren, in the absence of biological parents from the household.

Our finding that married grandmothers reported feeling psychosocial distress less frequently than their non-married counterparts is consistent with previous studies reporting that individuals who are married or have a partner report lower rates of depressive symptoms, relative to those without a partner (Penninx, Beekman, Ormel, Kriegsman, Boeke, & vanEijk, 1998). The positive effect of being married or having a partner may be partially explained by the adaptation process and family stress theory. Although we did not have a measure of relationship quality, and the data did not allow us to examine whether or to what extent the husbands and partners provided caregiving assistance to the grandmothers, adaptation strategies and efforts to minimize the stress of providing care for the grandchildren are plausible explanations (Brandon, 2000); and we presume that the positive benefits of marriage/partnering found in our study can be attributed to the help and support received by the grandmothers from their mates. Of course, it is not marriage per se, but the quality of the relationship that can strongly affect a person's emotional well-being (Gove, Hughes, & Style, 1983). A related finding was the positive effect of having other relatives living in the household. Similar to the positive benefits of having a spouse or partner, having relatives living in the household may likely contribute to the successful adaptation of the family, and contribute to the caregiving and support of the grandchild.

It is no surprise that not receiving welfare payments for childcare, or having a family income below the poverty level (e.g., severely poor or near poor) were associated with more frequent feelings of emotional distress. One serious consequence of becoming a custodial grandparent is a change for the worse in the grandparent's financial status (Mullen, 1996). Previous investigations have shown that the majority of custodial grandparents reported having less money than before they assumed custody; and that their current incomes were inadequate to meet their grandchildren's needs (Jendrek, 1993; Burton, 1992; Minkler & Roe, 1993). One reasonable explanation for the positive effect of not receiving welfare is that under the present welfare structure Temporary Assistance to Needy Family (TANF) has work requirements, time limits, and other restrictions that may be difficult to manage for many grandmother caregivers. These requirements may constrain a low-income grandparent's ability to receive benefits for her family, and thus exacerbate an already difficult economic situation.

Our findings indicated that almost 68% of the grandmothers had family incomes in the severely poor to near poor range. Minkler (1999) points out the historic differences in the level of aid afforded widowed mothers versus mothers who were single as a result of non-marriage, divorce, or desertion, and later between foster care and Aid to Families with Dependent Children. She notes the controversy over whether grandmothers are more "deserving" of aid than single mothers, or foster parents, for that matter. The welfare reform of 1996 continues this historical inequity and selectivity and fuels the controversy over who is deserving of public assistance. Many grandparent caregivers from low-income families encounter difficulties in obtaining public assistance and making ends meet. For example, Temporary Assistance for Needy Families (TANF) funds cannot be used to provide assistance to a family that includes an adult who has received such assistance for 60 months. Any previous use as first-generation parents counts against the caregiving grandparent by restricting the duration of their eligibility for public assistance (Caputo, 2000). Furthermore, the majority of grandchildren of younger caregiving grandparents are most likely co-residing with their grandchildren for three or more years and a considerable number do so for five or more years (Caputo, 2000). A grandmother might want to work rather than receive welfare, but for those without a husband or partner who could provide childcare or work more himself, increasing her hours of work is difficult (Brandon, 2000).

It is interesting that grandparents who reported having a usual place for health care also reported more emotional distress. Intuitively, we might have anticipated that having a usual place for health care would facilitate better care for the grandchild, thus, less emotional distress. However, although somewhat speculative, a plausible explanation is that this finding might be due to the stress of having to interact more frequently with a health care system that does nothing to eliminate the complexity or make it easier for caregiving grandparents to obtain health care for their grandchild. For example, grandparents may need legal authority to get their grandchildren medical care, and to enable them to receive immunizations and vaccinations, public assistance, and supportive services (Administration on Aging, 2000). Also, as pointed out by Weigers and colleagues (1998), many "usual care" providers do not have office hours that are convenient, or are often difficult to contact. More research into this aspect of the context social support of skipped generation households is warranted. Qualitative research would be especially useful in understanding the meaning of, and satisfaction with access to health care for this population of grandparent caregivers.

In considering the importance of regional differences in the context of skipped generation households, Model 4 suggests several questions for future research. For example, in the Midwest, why do the "women's issues" (e.g., being poor and female; or being Black and female) produce such disparate outcomes? For example, overall, what is it about living in the Midwest compared to other regions of the United States that diminishes the negative effect of poverty on psychosocial distress for skipped generation grandmothers? One answer might be that the comparatively small proportion of poor people, less stressful lifestyle, and less debasing access to public support make being poor more tenable, compared to other regions of the country. Yet, for Black grandmothers living in the Midwest, these same positive socioenvironmental factors produce strikingly opposite outcomes. It is reasonable to consider that in part, among Black skipped generation grandmothers living in the Midwest the greater frequency of feeling psychosocial distress might be attributed to social isolation, alienation, and the loss of important life roles, such as "traditional" (non-custodial) grandparenting, leisure pursuits, and free time (Kelly, 1983). Unfortunately, from these data, there is no way to test this proposed theory. Therefore, it is imperative that researchers conduct national qualitative studies looking at the subjective meaning of being a skipped generation grandparent with an eye towards uncovering regional distinctions.

CONCLUSION

Despite the obvious benefits of a national probability sample, these data are limited in that they only considered at most, one grandchild per family in each age cohort (0-5; 6-17). Consequently, we were unable to determine whether the number of grandchildren being cared for in the home influenced the grandparent's psychosocial distress in any way. Another limitation of this study is that the measure of psychosocial distress is not comparable to other standard measures of depression such as the Center for Epidemiological Studies Depression Scale (CES-D) (Radloff, 1977). As a result, we were unable to make any assessment of an appropriate cut-score that would indicate a risk for clinical depression, or to adequately compare the level of psychosocial distress to other studies of depression among older adults. Undertaking the care of a grandchild is associated with a significant increase in the level of psychosocial distress. The importance of psychological counseling for these grandparents is clear. As others have already recommended, social services and health providers can play an important role in helping these grandmothers to overcome barriers, such as fear of stigma, financial cost, or lack of information about available services (Minkler, Fuller-Thompson, Miller, & Driver, 2000)

It is apparent that more favorable consideration must be given to public assistance for caregiving grandparents especially to poor women who are more likely to be the caregivers in skipped generation households. It is imperative that more policy makers acknowledge the social good accomplished by these women caregivers, who are struggling to keep their families intact, despite incredible barriers. An exemption from the welfare-related time limit is a starting point to assisting the skipped generation grandparents, who, for the most part, are truly disadvantaged.

REFERENCES

Administration on Aging (2000). Grandparents Raising Grandchildren. Online [available] http://www.aoa.dhhs.gov/factsheets/grandparents.html

Brandon, P. (2000). Welfare Entries Among Children Living with Grandparents. *In JCPR Working Papers from Northwestern University/University of Chicago Joint Center for Poverty Research*. Online [available]: http://econpapers.hhs.se/paper/wopjopovw/170.htm.

Brogan, D.J. (1998). *Pitfalls of using standard statistical software for survey data*. In P. Armitage and T. Colton (Eds.), *Encyclopedia of biostatistics*. New York: John Wiley. Online [available]. http://www.fas.harvard.edu/~stats/survey-soft/donna_brogan. html

Bryson, K. & Casper, L.M. (1999). *Coresident grandparents and grandchildren*. U.S. Department of Commerce, Current Population Reports, P23-198.

Burnette, D. (1999). Custodial grandparents in Latino families: Patterns of service use and predictors of unmet needs. *Social Work, 44*, 22-34.

Burton, L. (1992). Black grandparents rearing children of drug-addicted parents: Stressors, outcomes, and social needs. *The Gerontologist, 32*, 744-751.

Caputo, R.K. (2001). Grandparents and coresident grandchildren in a youth cohort. *Journal of Family Issues, 22*, 541-556.

Caputo, R.K. (2000). Second-generation parenthood: A panel study of grandmother and grandchild coresidency among low-income families, 1967-1992. *Journal of Sociology and Social Welfare, 27(3)*, 3-20.

Casper, L., & Bryson, K. (1998). Co-resident grandparents and their grandchildren: Grandparent maintained families. *Population Division Working Paper No. 26*, Population Division, Bureau of the Census, Washington, DC.

Chalfie, D. (1994). *Going it alone: A closer look at grandparents parenting grandchildren.* Washington, DC: American Association for Retired Persons.

Fuller-Thompson, E. & Minkler, M. (2000). African American grandparents raising grandchildren: A national profile of demographic and health characteristics. *Health & Social Work 25*, 109-118.

Fuller-Thompson, E., Minkler, M., & Driver, D. (1997). A profile of grandparents raising grandchildren in the United States. *The Gerontologist, 37*, 406-411.

Giarrusso, R., Feng, D., Wang, Q., & Silverstein, M. (1996). "Parenting and co-parenting of grand-children": Effects on grandparents' well-being and family solidarity. *The International Journal of Sociology and Social Policy 16*(12), 124-154.

Gove, W., Hughes, M., & Style, C. (1983). Does marriage have positive effects on the well-being of the individual? *Journal of Health and Social Behavior, 24*, 122-131.

Goodman, C.C. & Silverstein, M. (2001). Grandmothers who parent their grandchildren: An exploratory study of close relations across three generations. *Journal of Family Issues 22*, 557-578.

Harrison, K.A., Richman, G.S., & Vittimberga, G.L. (2000). Parental stress in grandparents versus parents raising children with behavioral problems. *Journal of Family Issues, 21*, 262-270.

Jendrek, M.P. (1993). Grandparents who parent their grandchildren: Effects on lifestyle. *Journal of Marriage and Family, 55*, 609-621.

Kelly, S.J., Yorker, B.C., & Whitley, D. (1997). To grandmother's house we go . . . and stay. Children raised in intergenerational families. *Journal of Gerontological Nursing, 23*(9), 12-20.

Kelly, S.J. (1993). Caregiver stress in grandparents raising grandchildren. *Journal of Nursing Scholarship, 25*, 331-336.

Mills, T.L. (2001). Grandparents and grandchildren: Shared lives, well-being, and institutional forces influencing intergenerational relationships. *Journal of Family Issues, 22*, 677-679.

Minkler, M. & Fuller-Thompson, E. (1999). The health of grandparents raising grandchildren: Results of a national study. *American Journal of Public Health 89*, 1384-1392.

Minkler, M., Fuller-Thompson, E., Miller, D., & Driver, D. (2000). Grandparent caregiving and depression. In B. Hayslip, Jr. & R. Goldberg-Glen (Eds.), *Grandparents raising grandchildren: Theoretical, empirical, and clinical perspectives* (pp. 207-219). New York: Springer.

Minkler, M. (1999). Intergenerational households headed by grandparents: Contexts, realities, and implications for policy. *Journal of Aging Studies, 13*, 199-218.

Minkler, M. & Roe, K. (1993). *Grandmothers as caregivers: Raising children of the crack cocaine epidemic.* Newbury Park, CA: Sage.

Mullen, F. (1996). Public benefits: Grandparents, grandchildren, and welfare reform. *Generations, 20*, 61-65.

National Committee to Preserve Social Security and Medicare (1998). *Statistics for grandparents raising grandchildren.* Online [available]: http://www.egyptianaaa.org/G-Statistics.htm

NSAF (1999a). *National survey of America's families public use file user's guide, Methodology Report No. 11.* Online [available]. The Urban Institute Web site: http://newfederalism.urban.org/nsaf

NSAF (1999b). *National survey of America's families focal child codebook.* Online [available]. The Urban Institute Web site: http://newfederalism.urban.org/nsaf

Nunnally, J.C. (1978). *Psychometric theory* (2nd ed). New York: McGraw-Hill.

Pebley, A.R. & Rudkin, L.L. (1999). Grandparents caring for grandchildren. *Journal of Family Issues 20,* 218-242.

Penninx, B.W.H.J., Beekman, A.T.F., Ormel, J., Kriegsman, D.M.W., Boeke, A.J.P., & van Eijk, J. Th. M. (1998). Effects of social support and personal coping resources on depressive symptoms: Different for various chronic diseases? *Health Psychology, 17,* 551-558.

Pinson-Milburn, N.M. & Fabian, E.S. (1996). Grandparents raising grandchildren. *Journal of Counseling & Development 74,* 548-554.

Pruchno, R. & McKenney, D. (2002). Psychological well-being of black and white grandmothers raising grandchildren: Examination of a two-factor model. *Journals of Gerontology, Series B: Psychological Sciences and Social Sciences, 57,* P444-P452.

Radloff, L.S. (1977). The CES-D scale: A self-report depression scale for researching the general population. *Applied Psychological Measurement, 1,* 385-401.

Roe, K.M. & Minkler, M. (1999). Grandparents raising grandchildren: Challenges and responses. *Generations 22* (4): 25-32.

Sands, R.G. & Goldberg-Glen, R.S. (2000). Factors associated with stress among grandparents raising their grandchildren. *Family Relations 49*(1), 97-105.

Sorensen, A. & McLanahan, S. (1990). Women's economic dependency and men's support obligations: Economic relations within households. In H. Becker (Ed.), *Life histories and generations,* vol. 1. (pp. 115-144). Utrecht, The Netherlands: University of Utrecht.

Stata Statistical Software (n.d.). Stata Corporation, College Station, TX.

U.S. Census (1999). *Embargoed report: Nearly 5.5 million children live with grandparents.* U.S. Department of Commerce News Release. Online [available]. www.census.gov/ Press-Release/1999/cb99-115.html

U.S. Census (2000). *Economic living arrangements of children: Household studies.* U.S. Department of Commerce Current Population Reports: P70-74.

Weigers, M.E., Weinick, R.M., & Cohen, J.W. (1998). Children's health, 1996. MEPS chartbook No. 1. Agency for Health Care Policy and Research. Online [available]: http://www.ahcpr.gov/research/chrtbk1/chrtbk1b.htm

Index

BOOK ORDER FORM!

Order a copy of this book with this form or online at:
http://www.haworthpress.com/store/product.asp?sku=5555

Challenges of Aging on U.S. Families
Policy and Practice Implications

____ in softbound at $29.95 ISBN-13: 978-0-7890-2877-8. / ISBN-10: 0-7890-2877-8.
____ in hardbound at $49.95 ISBN-13: 978-0-7890-2876-1. / ISBN-10: 0-7890-2876-X.

COST OF BOOKS ____

POSTAGE & HANDLING ____
US: $4.00 for first book & $1.50
for each additional book
Outside US: $5.00 for first book
& $2.00 for each additional book.

SUBTOTAL ____
In Canada: add 7% GST. ____

STATE TAX ____
CA, IL, IN, MN, NJ, NY, OH, PA & SD residents
please add appropriate local sales tax.

FINAL TOTAL ____
If paying in Canadian funds, convert
using the current exchange rate,
UNESCO coupons welcome.

❏ BILL ME LATER:
Bill-me option is good on US/Canada/
Mexico orders only; not good to jobbers,
wholesalers, or subscription agencies.

❏ Signature ____

❏ Payment Enclosed: $ ____

❏ PLEASE CHARGE TO MY CREDIT CARD:
❏ Visa ❏ MasterCard ❏ AmEx ❏ Discover
❏ Diner's Club ❏ Eurocard ❏ JCB

Account # ____

Exp Date ____

Signature ____
(Prices in US dollars and subject to change without notice.)

PLEASE PRINT ALL INFORMATION OR ATTACH YOUR BUSINESS CARD

Name

Address

City   State/Province   Zip/Postal Code

Country

Tel   Fax

E-Mail

May we use your e-mail address for confirmations and other types of information? ❏ Yes ❏ No We appreciate receiving
your e-mail address. Haworth would like to e-mail special discount offers to you, as a preferred customer.
We will never share, rent, or exchange your e-mail address. We regard such actions as an invasion of your privacy.

Order from your **local bookstore** or directly from
The Haworth Press, Inc. 10 Alice Street, Binghamton, New York 13904-1580 • USA
Call our toll-free number (1-800-429-6784) / Outside US/Canada: (607) 722-5857
Fax: 1-800-895-0582 / Outside US/Canada: (607) 771-0012
E-mail your order to us: orders@haworthpress.com

For orders outside US and Canada, you may wish to order through your local
sales representative, distributor, or bookseller.
For information, see http://haworthpress.com/distributors

(Discounts are available for individual orders in US and Canada only, not booksellers/distributors.)

The Haworth Press, Inc.

Please photocopy this form for your personal use.
www.HaworthPress.com

BOF05